CDI Workbook:
Investigating Complex Cases and Formulating Queries

Sheila Duhon, MBA, RN, CCDS, A-CCRN, CCS

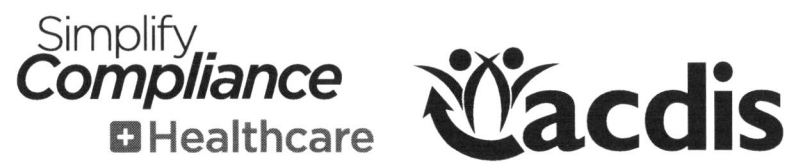

CDI Workbook: Investigating Complex Cases and Formulating Queries is published by HCPro, an H3.Group division of Simplify Compliance LLC.

Copyright © 2018 HCPro, an H3.Group division of Simplify Compliance LLC.

All rights reserved. Printed in the United States of America.   5   4   3   2   1

ISBN: 978-1-68308-806-6

No part of this publication may be reproduced, in any form or by any means, without prior written consent of HCPro or the Copyright Clearance Center (978-750-8400). Please notify us immediately if you have received an unauthorized copy.

HCPro provides information resources for the healthcare industry. HCPro is not affiliated in any way with The Joint Commission, which owns the JCAHO and Joint Commission trademarks.

Sheila Duhon, MBA, RN, CCDS, A-CCRN, CCS, Author
Linnea Archibald, Editor
Rebecca Hendren, Product Manager
Erin Callahan, Vice President, Product Development and Content Strategy
Elizabeth Petersen, President, H3.Group
Matt Sharpe, Senior Manager of Production
Vincent Skyers, Design Services Director
Mike Mirabello, Layout/Graphic Design
Mike King, Cover Designer

Advice given is general. Readers should consult professional counsel for specific legal, ethical, or clinical questions. Arrangements can be made for quantity discounts. For more information, contact:

HCPro
35 Village Road, Suite 200
Middleton, MA 01949
Telephone: 800-650-6787 or 781-639-1872
Fax: 800-639-8511
Email: *customerservice@hcpro.com*

Visit HCPro online at *www.hcpro.com* and *www.hcmarketplace.com*

Table of Contents

Introduction vii

Chapter 1: Clinical Documentation Improvement Program Practices and Competencies 1

    Historical Perspective 1
    Mission Statement 3
    Steering Committee 5
    Organizational Reporting Structure 5
    Hiring and Training New CDI Specialists 7
    Measurements of Success 9
    The Value of a Robust CDI Program 12

Chapter 2: Physician Engagement and Education 15

    A Comprehensive Team Approach 15
    The CDI Specialist 16
    The Physician Provider 17
    Engaging Physicians 18
    The Physician Advisor 22
    The Physician Advisor's Role in CDI 24

Chapter 3: A Compliant Query Practice 29

    Historical Perspective 29
    Authoritative Guidance 30
        AHIMA 30

TABLE OF CONTENTS

ACDIS 31
The Health Insurance Portability and Accountability Act (HIPAA)
and the four Cooperating Parties 32
The False Claims Act and the Stark Law 33
The Query Process 34
AHIMA and ACDIS joint brief, 2016 34
The AHIMA 6 34
What is a leading query? 35
What is a compliant query? 36
Query Storage and Retrieval 37
The verbal query versus the written query 37
There Is No Correct or Incorrect Response to a Query 38
The Concurrent Query Process 39
The Retrospective Query Process 39
When a Provider Refuses to Respond to a Query 40
Authorized Persons Who Can Query a Provider 40
The Query Format 41
Open-ended queries 41
Multiple-choice queries 42
Yes/no queries 43
Writing Effective Queries: Best Practices 44
The "TRIC" to query success 44
The "dos" for an effective query process 46
The "don'ts" for an effective query process 46

Chapter 4: Case Studies: Exercises in the Practical Application of the CDI Review Process 49

Tips for Reviewing the Case Studies 49
Case Study: Neurology 51
Case Study: Hematology 59
Case Study: Cardiovascular 65
Case Study: Nephrology 71
Case Study: Procedures 76
Case Study: Nutrition 83
Case Study: Multiple Conditions 92
Case Study: Neoplastic Disease 112

Chapter 5: Leading and Managing a CDI Program 127

CDI Program Evolution 127
CDI Program Leadership 128
CDI Program Management 129
    Prioritization of reviews 130
    Distribution of reviews 131
    Provisional coding 132
    CDI specialist development 133
    Measurement of CDI program goals 134
The Big Data, the Little Data, and the "Intangible" Data 135
Conclusion 138

Introduction

Chances are pretty good that if you've purchased this book or have been assigned to study this practical guide, you are committed to strengthening your clinical documentation integrity (CDI) skills and foundational CDI knowledge. The professional CDI specialist (commonly referred to as the CDIS, CDS, or CDI professional) must possess a wide swath of proficiency that includes sound and solid clinical expertise, more than a passing knowledge of coding guidelines and rules, a hearty dose of determination and perseverance, an abundance of interpersonal skills that can seamlessly cross multitudes of personalities, and, perhaps most importantly, a keen sense of ethics that is above reproach.

The information and guidance provided in this book are designed to assist you in strengthening your overall CDI skills, but most specifically in the area of record review and query development. As you proceed through the chapters in this workbook, you will gain a better understanding of the foundation of the CDI review process. You will be challenged with case scenarios that will likely generate thoughtful discussion, perhaps differences of opinion, and finally a renewed appreciation for the critical analysis of all components of the medical decision-making that comes into play for each and every record a CDI specialist reviews.

We approach this goal through a robust dive into case studies and opportunities for gleaning further specificity and accuracy in the medical record that is reflective of the true severity of illness, risk of mortality, and intensity of resources expended to care for all the relevant diagnoses the patient has during the encounter for care. The ultimate goal for the CDI review is that the final coded medical record is reflective of the clinical truth, with the integrity of the final coded data above reproach and scrutiny for any misrepresentation or inaccuracies.

Given the significance of ensuring the integrity of the final coded record, it might be a bit surprising to realize that CDI specialists are relatively new on the healthcare scene, with their origins only reaching

INTRODUCTION

back about a decade or a little more. The emergence of the CDI profession has developed as a result of increasingly more complex diagnoses and procedures, coding and billing requirements and practices, regulatory and governing bodies that demand documentation be aligned with scientific evidence-based standards of care, and public expectation for accountability by the healthcare profession to report all aspects of care delivery and outcomes with transparency and accuracy.

The Association of Clinical Documentation Improvement Specialists (ACDIS) was developed from the need to establish a professional body that stood to define, guide, and navigate the emergence of this new profession within healthcare. In addition to your own program's educational efforts, I encourage CDI professionals to embrace the opportunities afforded through active engagement with the learning that ACDIS offers, both at the local ACDIS chapter level and at the national level. There are numerous publications offered, free of charge to the CDI community at large. *ACDIS Radio* is offered free on a biweekly basis and is an excellent source of information and updates affecting the CDI profession. Other resources are offered through membership in the organization. Whichever way you may choose to participate, the knowledge gained will empower you and strengthen your skills as a CDI professional. So, don't hold back—go for it! You will be glad you did!

Happy learning!

Sheila Duhon, MBA, RN, CCDS, A-CCRN, CCS
National director of CDI education at Tenet Healthcare
Dallas, Texas

CHAPTER 1
Clinical Documentation Improvement Program Practices and Competencies

Historical Perspective

Clinical documentation improvement (CDI) programs were originally borne from an effort to optimize the documentation in the medical record, allowing the coders to capture the best possible Medicare Severity Diagnosis-Related Group (MS-DRG) for each patient. This process was (and still is) achieved through physicians' documentation of comorbid conditions (CC) and major CCs (MCC). CDI specialists were trained to recognize the CCs and MCCs that the providers were not capturing in the documentation within the clinical record.

When something appeared to be missing, incomplete, or confusing in the documentation, the CDI specialist would query the provider for more specific diagnoses that would in turn drive the DRG to a higher-weighted, longer length of stay (LOS) and ultimately a higher reimbursement level than would have been assigned before the query. Those improvements were concurrently reflected in a higher case-mix index (CMI) for the organization as a whole. (We'll discuss coding nuances off and on throughout this book.)

Since those straightforward beginnings, CDI programs have changed dramatically. Over the past decade or more, CDI programs have increasingly focused on ensuring a clear, concise, compliant, and complete medical record for more than simply financial reimbursement optimization. CDI programs have a footprint in many areas of an organization, including but not limited to:

- Quality assessment
- Utilization management
- Organization public profiles

CHAPTER 1

- Medical staff public profiles
- Financial forecasting
- Resource allocation
- Clinical care
- Data-driven indicators such as:
  - CMI
  - Severity of illness
  - Risk of mortality
  - Length of stay

Utilizing the data is key to assessing performance, recognizing opportunities for process improvement, identifying outliers, and tracking trends. An organization that assesses the data month to month will have greater insights into performance on many levels. Consequently, greater financial health of the organization will ensure the organization's mission to serve and care for its community members is met. (Data and metrics will be discussed further in Chapter 5.)

Many programs have even gone so far as to change the title of the program from clinical documentation improvement to clinical documentation integrity to emphasize the heightened focus on integrity and clinical truth in the medical record. Clear, concise, compliant, and complete documentation, every single time in every single record, is the cornerstone for achieving that end. That's where CDI makes an indelible mark.

Over the years, the CDI profession has seen astoundingly immense growth in a relatively short period of time. In the beginning, there were just a few small programs that were born of the desire to "capture the correct DRG." In 2008, The Association of Clinical Documentation Improvement Specialists (ACDIS) held its first annual conference in Las Vegas with just more than 500 attendees. That same conference now attracts thousands of attendees annually.

Additionally, there are now several certifications offered specifically for those in the CDI profession, the first being the Certified Clinical Documentation Specialist (CCDS) credential offered through ACDIS. As of the writing of this book, more than 4,000 people hold an active CCDS credential. The world of CDI is dynamic and constantly morphing into expanded roles and impact across the organization.

Mission Statement

A successful CDI program must begin with a clearly defined end goal that is articulated in a mission statement. The scope, intent, and impact of the program are internally driven by the stakeholders within the organization. Each stakeholder should understand and wholly support the goals, intent, and potential impact. Typical stakeholders for a CDI program include the CDI specialist, the CDI program leadership, the organizational senior leadership, and physicians. Ancillary departments often have a stake in the mission of CDI as well, though, including case management, quality, business/revenue cycle, legal, and compliance, among others.

When developing a mission statement, it's advisable to form a steering committee including the relevant stakeholders mentioned previously. This ensures that all the invested parties support and approve of the program's mission and understand how the CDI program fits into the larger organizational mission. For existing programs without a clear and current mission statement, consider raising the concern during an upcoming administrative meeting and incorporating the statement into the existing CDI policies and procedures.

Without a clearly articulated mission statement, the organization risks deviating from the original intent of the program. A mission statement need not be extensive or verbose. It must simply state the intent, process, and anticipated outcomes of the program. An example of a clear mission statement is:

> *The CDI program exists to ensure that clear, concise, compliant, and complete documentation in the medical record accurately reflects the true condition of the patient, reflective of the severity of illness (SOI), risk of mortality (ROM) and the intensity of services (IOS) necessary to care for the patient. Concurrent collaboration with the physician provider will ensure the most precise codes are assigned to the encounter for care, contributing to accurate data collection, outcome measurement, and appropriate reimbursement.*

It's also important to remember that simply because a CDI program began its life with a specific mission statement does not preclude that mission from evolving over time. As the program matures, additional

CHAPTER 1

themes may be added to the mission statement to address specific issues as they arise. For example, establishing a cohesive communication line between clinical and coding staffs might be an appropriate addition for a facility that traditionally struggles with cross-department dialogue.

Considering how dynamic the CDI world is, an annual review of the CDI mission statement serves as an opportunity to update and add new scope to the program. All the original stakeholders should be involved in an annual review, as well as any new stakeholders, as the scope of the original program expands and becomes more diverse.

The mission statement should also influence the everyday policies and procedures employed by the CDI program. Policies should generally include the scope of coverage, the purpose of the policy, any definitions included in the policy, and lastly the specific policy guidelines that govern the practices and expectations of the team responsible for operating within the policy.

Policy and procedure development should align with industry standards. The Centers for Medicare & Medicaid Services (CMS), ACDIS, and the American Health Information Management Association (AHIMA) are each highly regarded as standard bearers for CDI. CDI program directors and managers should review their respective resources when developing policies and procedures to ensure they remain compliant and up to date.

Though often stated together as "policies and procedures," it is important to note that a policy is much different from a procedure. A policy is a document that states the general rules, principles, and guidelines developed by the stakeholders within an organization that will serve to achieve the overarching goals. Specifics within a policy can include the mission statement of the program and identify the stakeholders, the established goals, and desired outcomes that can be tracked as measures of success of the program.

A procedure, on the other hand, is a document and should include reference to a policy and provide specific action steps that are required to ensure compliance with the policy. Procedures address more specific operational expectations, platforms, and directives on workflow processes. A procedure is more specific in the day-to-day operations and functions required to reach the mission stated in the policy. For example, when new technology is introduced, the daily operating procedure may change as a result. The procedure should be kept current with the actual workflow process.

Steering Committee

Often, a CDI program's mission is governed by a steering committing consisting of the major stakeholders from departments affected by the CDI program's focus. These departments may include:

- Compliance
- Medical staff
- Revenue cycle
- Case management
- Health information management (HIM)/coding
- Executive leadership
- Clinical quality

In order to reach the desired mission of the CDI program and support the overall organizational goals, it is crucial to include leadership from these key areas when discussing the goals of the CDI program. No department is an island, so ensure that the CDI program contributes to the overall goals of the organization. Additionally, including leadership and stakeholders in the development of the mission statement ensures their commitment to the success of the CDI program and acknowledges the value the program brings to the stakeholders and the organization as a whole.

Members of the steering committee can each apply their different training, unique insights, and job experiences to the task of CDI program organization. For example, if coders are held to productivity benchmarks, the HIM director may want to develop a process by which CDI staff contact the coding supervisor rather than individual coders to avoid interrupting the workflow process of an individual coder. This serves to provide CDI specialists with a resource to turn to when coding questions arise, yet still allows that overall goals for productivity are secure.

Organizational Reporting Structure

The organizational reporting structure for a CDI program often derives directly from the mission statement. If the core focus of the program is documentation integrity, the most common organizational structure follows the HIM reporting model. ACDIS demonstrated the following results from the 2017 CDI Salary Survey, an annual survey conducted over the past four consecutive years:

CDI DEPARTMENT REPORTING STRUCTURE

	2014	2015	2016	2017
Case management	20.5%	16%	14.3%	11.24%
Chief financial officer	10.4%	11.4%	13.7%	11.62%
Chief medical officer	2.2%	3%	2.6%	2.5%
CDI manager/director	17.7%	25.1%	18.4%	19.88%
HIM manager/director	39.9%	34.2%	31.9%	34.77%
Quality manager/director	9.3%	10.2%	8.1%	8.26%
Other	N/A	N/A	11%	11.72%

Source: 2017 CDI Salary Survey, ACDIS.

The year-over-year trend reflects a movement away from case management (and, to a slightly lesser degree, away from the quality department) to a stronger emphasis of placing CDI in a HIM department or a separate and independent CDI model.

This trend in CDI reporting might naturally reflect the effect and focus for CDI having a pure commitment to clear, concise, compliant, and complete documentation every single time in every single record, regardless of impact on case management, quality measures, or reimbursement outcomes. There exists a potential for bias and mission creep when CDI is within a department that has more than one mission. Though many organizations work well with placing CDI in the quality, case management, or even revenue cycle departments, extra caution must be exercised to avoid the potential pitfalls of bias or mission creep.

Ultimately, CDI should not serve many masters. Mission creep is a distinct possibility when CDI programs are directed to serve multiple functions across the organization in an attempt to ensure revenue, quality scoring, and justification for increased LOS. Rather, a single focus of the clinical truth in the documentation in the medical record should be the mission of the CDI program. All medical record reviews, conversations with providers, and queries should be prompted by that single focus for truth and integrity of the final coded record.

For example, shouldn't accurate documentation automatically reflect present-on-admission (POA) indicators? With complete and accurate documentation, the medical record should already ensure that quality data accurately reflects which conditions were POA versus which conditions the patient acquired during the hospital encounter. Identification of conditions acquired during the hospital encounter may reflect poorly on facility quality scoring, yet it will ultimately drive process and care improvement. Isn't that what we all strive for—the best quality care each and every time for each and every patient we serve, regardless of reporting structure?

Hiring and Training New CDI Specialists

The CDI specialist is undoubtedly the most crucial piece of the puzzle when forming a new CDI program or expanding an existing one. A CDI specialist is a uniquely qualified individual and, as such, this is not a career path for the faint of heart or for those who view the role as a reward for service in the acute care clinical setting, one step closer to retirement. When building a CDI program and CDI specialists from the ground up, there are some required qualities leaders should look for in order to place the most qualified person in a CDI specialist role. The CDI team comprised of a balanced mix of backgrounds is often the strongest team in terms of skill set and impact.

The job of a CDI specialist is not merely an office job that requires reviewing the medical record with the occasional query for clarification to obtain a CC or MCC for coding and reimbursement purposes. CDI has progressed far beyond the early days of maximizing the DRG for optimal reimbursement and CMI, as discussed previously. CDI professionals need to have a strong clinical and coding background, combined with the critical-thinking skills to investigate a record closely and put the "clinical puzzle" together. Additionally, CDI specialists must possess strong interpersonal skills in order to communicate with and educate physicians.

We'll discuss more of the specific requirements for a CDI professional in Chapter 2, but for now, let's talk a bit about hiring the right CDI professional. A truly qualified CDI specialist is a master of many skills, including:

- Clinical acumen
- Coding knowledge

CHAPTER 1

- Critical thinking
- Data analysis
- Time management
- Ability to adapt to changing workflow processes and platforms
- Exceptional interpersonal skills to relate to clinicians and operational teams fluently
- Computer and software skills

Complicating things further, the CDI specialist needs to be able to use all these skills in both face-to-face and electronic communications.

This is not an easy or common combination to find. As such, the individuals meeting the specific criteria are often in high demand and the shortage of truly qualified individuals dictates that some organizations "grow their own" CDI specialists in order to fill the gap. Many organizations mentor highly skilled clinicians or advanced HIM/coding professionals and teach the CDI process and skills by means of on-the-job training, internally sponsored computer-based curricula, boot camps, or a combination of these approaches and more.

According to the 2017 Salary Survey from ACDIS, the most common background for a CDI specialist by far is clinical, and most often from a registered nursing background. The majority of this population is female, with nearly 85% being at least 40 years old.

CDI specialists who come to the profession from a strictly coding background and those who come from a foreign-educated physician background comprise the second-most-populous groups of CDI specialists in the United States, according to the survey.

Combining the appropriate clinical and coding foundational background with the right personality is the key to finding the best, and ultimately the most successful, CDI specialist. Optimal CDI specialist performance equals CDI program success; therefore, it is in the best interest of the CDI leadership team to match the right person with the right role.

Even a CDI specialist with superb clinical or coding knowledge, however, may not be the best fit for the role if the ability to interact with physicians and other providers is not a strength the CDI specialist possesses. A CDI specialist needs to have a degree of resilience and must expect a fair amount of pushback from providers who do not fully understand the intent of the CDI program. A CDI specialist who can withstand the challenge from providers and rationally demonstrate the intent of the CDI process is truly invaluable to the overall program's success. In order to succeed, CDI specialists need to understand that providers ultimately want what is best for the patient. Pairing accurate documentation with the care provided is the best outcome for all involved, most importantly the patient. (A more in-depth discussion regarding physician engagement and education is included in Chapter 2.)

The Joint Commission requires that specific documents reflecting the care and treatment of conditions for hospitalized patients be completed in a timely and accurate manner by the providers of care. It is a Joint Commission standard that a comprehensive history and physical be completed and entered into the official medical record within 24 hours of admission to the hospital.

Additionally, when applicable, a timely and complete operative procedure note must also be present in the medical record. Documents such as these present CDI specialists with the material from which to evaluate if clear, concise, compliant, and complete documentation exists in the record. If there are gaps in the documentation, or inconclusive, imprecise, unclear, or conflicting documentation present in the record, then the CDI specialist is required to submit a query to clarify the intent of the provider's documentation.

TIPS FOR DEVELOPING A MEDICAL RECORD REVIEW PROCESS

A brand-new CDI specialist may understandably feel a bit overwhelmed when they consider the history and scope of CDI's practice and the quantity of required knowledge. While each CDI specialist may have his or her own unique approach to conducting a record review, a new CDI staff member can learn immensely from more tenured teammates. Because of this, new CDI specialists should spend some time shadowing existing members whenever possible as part of their onboarding and training process.

Measurements of Success

After the CDI program is launched and the CDI specialists are off and running, program leaders need to evaluate and measure the success of the program. As evidenced by the history and evolution of CDI over the past decade or more, CDI is not a stagnant profession; therefore, a program cannot maintain success without assessing the program outcomes and impact for the organization over time. Metrics and assessment of the metrics may need to change and evolve to maintain relevancy.

CHAPTER 1

Program leaders and other stakeholders should assess the outcomes carefully to identify whether the CDI program's goals are being met or if those goals need to be amended to accommodate for new focus areas and institutional goals. The best practice is to assess alignment with the program's mission statement at least on a quarterly basis (though monthly would be even better) to ensure it still matches and is supported by the actual outcomes of the program. The more focus that is centered on a continual, monthly performance to achieve the program mission and goals, the timelier any intervention will be to support any areas noted as deficient.

Typical CDI program metrics may include:

- Trending and monitoring of overall patient volumes
- Service line fluctuations
- CC/MCC capture rate
- Relative weight changes
- CMI changes
- Geometric mean LOS (GMLOS) days
- Physician response to query rates
- Timeliness of physician responses to the query process
- DRG impact of physician response to queries
- Reimbursement impact from query responses
- SOI/ROM impact from query responses
- Mortality rates with incongruent SOI/ROM
- Hospital-acquired conditions (HAC)
- Patient safety indicators (PSI)
- Audit and denial rates

While these metrics are outcome-centered, CDI programs should also delve into their own internal metrics as well, with a more focused assessment of individual CDI specialists' performance. Ideally, monthly program metrics should be reported to all key stakeholders in alignment with the CDI program mission statement.

CLINICAL DOCUMENTATION IMPROVEMENT PROGRAM PRACTICES AND COMPETENCIES

Typical CDI specialist performance metrics may include:

- Medical record review rates

- Query rates

- Physician response to query rate

    - Physician "agreed" rate

    - Physician "disagreed" rate

    - Physician "no response" rate

- Quality and compliance of CDI specialists' queries

    - Appropriate and nonleading clinical indicators that are relevant to the focus of the query:

        - Treatment of the condition is relevant to the encounter

        - Risk of the condition is relevant to the encounter

        - Imprecise or lack of specificity of the condition may be relevant to the encounter

    - Appropriate formatting of the query: clear, concise, succinct, and professionally written

    - Query addressed to the appropriate physician

    - Nonleading question posed to the provider

- Compliance of the CDI specialist's queries with ethical and coding guidelines and AHIMA and ACDIS standards

- Missed documentation improvement opportunities (when a query wasn't presented to the provider that could have or should have been)

- Education presentations by the CDI specialist to the medical staff

- Collaboration from the CDI specialist with other hospital departments

- Collaboration of the CDI specialist with coding and HIM professionals

- Impact of CDI reviews and queries on organizational goals

    - Financial

CHAPTER 1

- Quality

- Utilization management

- Risk reduction

- Compliance

- Other organization-specific impact aligned with the mission statement for the organization

The Value of a Robust CDI Program

Ultimately, CDI is an essential element of an organization that strives to provide quality services to the population served. Value is the measurement of the outcomes of the services rendered in relation to the resources spent to provide those services. Terrance Govender, MD, vice president of medical affairs at ClinIntell, Inc., in Seattle, Washington, teaches this concept succinctly as:

$$Value = \frac{Quality}{Cost}$$

When assessing value, it's important to remember that stakeholders expect value delivered from all disciplines. The patient (consumer) places trust in the physician, the nursing and ancillary care staff, and the hospital as a whole. In turn, the physician, the nurses, and ancillary teams trust that the hospital will provide the resources, treatment modalities, medications, and equipment necessary for them to provide safe, effective, and efficient care to the patient. The hospital administration expects that the use of the resources provided to care for the patient are appropriately used and administered safely by competent and professional healthcare providers and that care is taken to avoid waste.

While there are many stakeholders expecting a CDI program to "prove its worth," so to speak, how a CDI program delivers that return on investment relies heavily on the stated mission. For example, a program with a focus on DRG optimization for financial purposes will likely demonstrate its worth through regular financial reporting. A program focusing on quality care measures, however, may provide stats from public reporting websites such as *Hospital Compare* from CMS.

A CDI program scope that includes the program metrics outlined in the preceding section will employ numerous sources and points of data to assess impact and value. Organizations that assess a multifaceted

CLINICAL DOCUMENTATION IMPROVEMENT PROGRAM PRACTICES AND COMPETENCIES

monthly dashboard are able to determine their effect at a comprehensive and high-level view and move forward with change and added value for all.

A CDI dashboard can contain several elements and points of focus. The following may serve as a beginning assessment of elements for inclusion and be further refined to reflect organizational mission and performance.

CDI dashboard elements and points of focus:

- Patient volume
    - Overall
    - Medical
    - Surgical
    - Service line volume
- GMLOS and actual LOS
- CMI
    - DRG migration
        - DRG with MCC
        - DRG with CC
        - DRG without MCC/CC
    - Migration from medical to surgical DRG
    - Case volume
- SOI/ROM
    - All Patient Refined-DRG migration
    - SOI/ROM migration
        - Principal diagnosis

CHAPTER 1

- Status and history codes

- Secondary diagnoses that are monitored, are treated, are evaluated, increase nursing care resources, and/or require an extended LOS

- Financial impact

  - May include the "obvious" and the "not so obvious"

    - Financial reimbursement from payer

    - Risk reduction for denial of payment or DRG downgrading

    - Efficiencies realized through accurate GMLOS assignment, congruent with the true clinical picture realized by accurate and precise documentation

    - Improved or maintained patient volume that may fluctuate with publicly reported data reflecting physician and hospital quality scores

REFERENCE

The Association of Clinical Documentation Improvement Specialists. (2018). *2017 Salary Survey: Salaries continue to grow, but participants are less optimistic than in the past* (Rep.). Middleton, MA: HCPro.

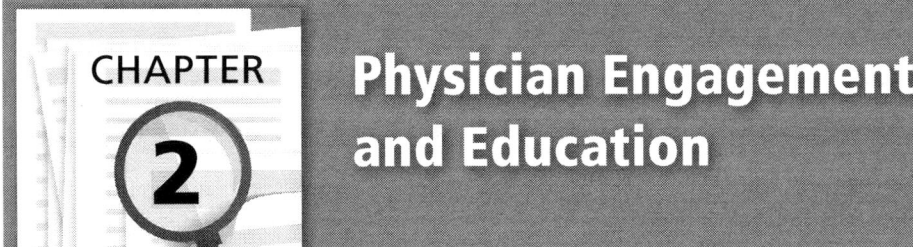

Physician Engagement and Education

A Comprehensive Team Approach

A successful clinical documentation improvement (CDI) program mandates cooperation and engagement from all stakeholders. The CDI team, in concert with coding, case management, clinical quality, compliance, revenue cycle, and the hospital executive team, must strive to engage medical staff leadership and the practicing medical staff members. This is sometimes easier said than done, requiring a solid and thoughtful approach to fostering engagement. Clear direction for coding integrity from both coding and care providers is given through the International Classification of Diseases, 10th edition (ICD-10), *Official Guidelines for Coding and Reporting*:

> *A joint effort between the healthcare provider and the coder is essential to achieve complete and accurate documentation, code assignment, and reporting of diagnoses and procedures. These guidelines have been developed to assist both the healthcare provider and the coder in identifying those diagnoses that are to be reported. The importance of consistent, complete documentation in the medical record cannot be overemphasized. Without such documentation, accurate coding cannot be achieved.*

Clearly, the directive here is that coding must accurately reflect the true clinical picture and course of care rendered throughout the hospital encounter. Given the reality that very few physicians are trained in the nuances of coding, this often presents a "disconnect" between the clinical side of the patient encounter and the coding/business side of the encounter, hence the need for the CDI specialist. The CDI specialist connects the dots and bridges the gap between physician's clinical language and coding language.

CHAPTER 2

The CDI Specialist

Successful CDI specialists are highly trained and clinically sound with a heightened sense of interpersonal and communication skills. According to the 2017 CDI Salary Survey from the Association of Clinical Documentation Improvement Specialists (ACDIS), 77% of respondents hold the registered nurse (RN) credential and have a strong clinical foundation gained from years of nursing in a variety of medical-surgical or specialty services.

This solid clinical acumen combined with critical analytic thinking skills provides a firm foundation upon which to add coding knowledge—and thus a CDI specialist is born. The CDI specialist who possesses sound clinical knowledge, demonstrates critical analysis thinking, exhibits the ability to collaborate with healthcare providers, and can "connect the dots" between the clinical world and the coding world is an invaluable asset to the organization and all its stakeholders.

The shift from a clinical perspective to a documentation and coding perspective is often a huge leap and requires education and training that involves a steep learning curve. ACDIS offers a Certified Clinical Documentation Specialist (CCDS) certification that requires a minimum of two full years of CDI experience before sitting for the exam. While this may seem like a rather long time period, it is actually reflective of the intense education and skills necessary to become a first-class CDI specialist, deserving of the distinction the CCDS credential represents.

Most CDI specialists need to learn the nuances of coding and the specificity required in documentation. Learning coding language is akin to learning a foreign language. This does not come naturally to most clinicians; therefore, CDI specialists coming from a clinical background undergo intense study consisting of but not necessarily limited to:

- Coding
- Major Diagnostic Categories (MDC)
- Diagnostic-Related Group (DRG) assignment
    - Medicare Severity-DRG (MS-DRG)
    - All Patient Refined-DRG (APR-DRG)
- American Health Information Management Association (AHIMA) guidelines
- Centers for Medicare & Medicaid Services (CMS) guidelines

- ACDIS guidelines
- Outcomes measurement
- Case-mix index (CMI)
- Length of stay (LOS)
- Severity of illness (SOI) assignment
- Risk of mortality (ROM) assignment
- Quality scoring
- Public data reporting
- Revenue cycle impact and forecasting
- Payment models
- Query development
- Medicare and regulatory agency requirements
- Ethical, legal, and compliance standards
- Provider engagement methods
- Risk reduction from audit and denials processes

Clearly, the accumulation of an entirely different and new skill set necessary for the CDI specialist requires dedication and commitment to grow in the CDI specialist role. This maturation process takes place over a period of months and even years.

The Physician Provider

A physician who understands the value of a CDI specialist is a physician who understands the changing dynamics of today's healthcare industry. Likewise, a physician who maintains an awareness of publicly reported data such as *Physician Compare* by CMS is better equipped to position themselves proactively for changes as they occur.

CDI specialists are often tasked with the responsibility to ensure the medical record contains clear, concise, legible, complete, reliable, and consistent documentation so that the final coded record is above reproach and is reflective of the true SOI, ROM, and intensity of services (IOS) rendered during the hospital encounter. To attain this end, the CDI specialist reviews the record in its entirety and submits a request for clarification when and if there is incomplete, inconsistent, unclear, illegible, inconsistent, imprecise, or unreliable documentation in the record. This request for clarification is submitted in the form of a query to the provider.

A query to the provider can be fraught with all sorts of problems if it is not well presented, focused, and relevant. Physicians are scientists whose focus is on patient care and outcomes. Coding is often viewed as a "game" of semantics: a nuisance and a wasteful, time-consuming part of their day that could be better spent caring for patients. Add to this scenario the mandates for electronic health record (EHR) participation, increased focus on discharging within the LOS allotted for the assigned DRG, regulatory requirements for medical necessity, demonstration of medical decision-making, among many other requirements, and it's easy to see why physicians are frustrated and may choose not to comply with documentation requests.

Engaging Physicians

It's clear that engaging and aligning providers with CDI efforts requires great finesse, skill, and understanding of the physician's perspective. Therefore, how do we engage and gain cooperation from medical staff? The best advice I have is to *know your message and be succinct, timely, and concise in delivering that message.* And, above all, *know and be present for your physicians.* Know them by sight and be present face-to-face or electronically to serve as a subject matter expert (SME), assisting them in documentation of the most accurate clinical picture, reflective of their medical decision-making expertise and interventions on behalf of the patient.

Let's look a bit deeper at each component of that advice:

- **Know your message:** Ask yourself what education you want to relay. What's the "disconnect" between what the physician documented (which, in his or her perspective, is entirely clear) and what the coding directive requires for specificity and correct code assignment?

- **Be succinct:** Physicians document their findings, assessments, plans, and impressions to communicate to other care providers. Physicians do not document to provide accurate code assignment. Therefore, when communicating with the physician (whether it be in a written or verbal form), be brief and to the point. Do not include information that is superfluous to the focus of the query. Stick only to the points that directly pertain to the query. Inclusion of past medical history and what brought the patient to the hospital may not be necessary when asking a physician who has attended to the patient for many years.

- **Be timely:** Choose the correct time to approach the physician. Be observant of the dynamics of the physician's behavior or demands on his or her time and attention at that moment. A physician who is handling an emergency clinical scenario is not likely to welcome a query about a different patient and topic at that moment. Submitting a query through an electronic platform can often circumvent the issue of timing. Electronic queries allow the physician to review the record and the query when it is most convenient for them.

- **Be concise:** Learn to deliver a succinct and focused message in a 30-second time frame. Practice this delivery, over and over again, out loud until you can state your message with confidence and credibility. Most physicians will give you 30 seconds to deliver a message; most will not give you five to 10 minutes to express the same message. Time is one of a physician's most valuable assets. Respect that and you will likely gain respect and cooperation in return.

- **Know and be present for your physician:** Be present on a regular basis for your physicians. Be sure you know the physician, by sight as well as name, and ensure the physician knows you by sight and name and your role. Daily interactions on the medical units foster a team-oriented and collaborative environment. Face-to-face communication is invaluable and cannot be conveyed in the same manner by phone, fax, or electronic medium. A collegial relationship that is fostered daily results in improved communication, participation, and outcomes for all stakeholders.

There no road maps that a CDI specialist can follow to avoid all the pitfalls along the way when mastering the fine art of communication with physicians. If only there was one! Don't despair, though. The "school of hard knocks" is often the best teacher, and I'll share some of the tips and techniques I have learned along the way with you.

I have the incredible honor to travel frequently across the country and engage with clinicians and CDI specialists from the east to the west coast, from the Canadian border to the Gulf of Mexico. Throughout my travels, the physicians and CDI specialists I engage with come from large complex teaching organizations, inner city hospitals, and tiny, small-town community hospitals. The stories shared and the experiences recounted to me make one thing crystal clear: the situations, successes, and obstacles we face as CDI specialists are a common thread in this tapestry we weave in the CDI world. So, how do we handle these challenges? First and foremost, keep a sense of humor! It's much easier to do that when I consider the life and death decisions and responsibility I shouldered every shift in the acute care hospital setting versus the more administrative responsibility I now shoulder in the CDI setting. Keep everything in perspective!

CHAPTER 2

Let me tell you a story I recall clearly from when I had about five years of CDI experience under my belt. I had just entered the medical intensive care unit (ICU) to round when Dr. Defiant (the names have been changed to protect all parties—innocent or otherwise) approached me right away and declared "I am NOT going to answer that query you left me about CHF [congestive heart failure]! You should ask the cardiologist, not me!" "Well," I thought to myself, "I would ask the cardiologist, but the cardiologist is not documenting anything about CHF. It is you, Dr. Defiant, that is the only physician on the case documenting CHF, which I agree, is not your specialty area."

So, how does one handle a situation like this—an angry physician declaring what he or she will or will not do, announcing it loudly, and in the middle of the nursing station? I chose the path of least resistance at that moment. I did not want to escalate or feed his anger, so I simply stated he had the choice to answer the query or not, and the reason I asked him the question was because I saw it in his documentation.

He grumbled a bit and we both went our separate ways within the ICU. About 20 minutes later, he came up to me, as he was on his way out of the ICU and said, "Hey, don't take that personally or anything." I smiled a huge smile inside: He clearly realized his declaration and behavior were a bit out of line. I answered him with a genuine smile and a bit of a laugh, "Dr. Defiant," I said, "I never take anything like that personally. I know that at the end of each day, I've done the best job I can do, and when I get home, my dog is happy to see me, my kids are happy to see me, my husband is happy to see me, and I will sleep well tonight." We parted ways on a bit of a lighter note that day. Smile.

The funny thing about that encounter is that Dr. Defiant and I had a really good working relationship before that incident and it continued after that incident. That little "blip" on the radar did not derail my mission as a CDI specialist and it did not deter him from responding to queries in the future. Oh, and did he ever answer that query? And if he did not, then who did? Ultimately, I deferred the query to the cardiologist, but not for clarification of the type, acuity, and etiology of the CHF. Rather, I asked whether the cardiologist agreed with Dr. Defiant's diagnosis of CHF. The cardiologist responded and clarified that the patient did not have a diagnosis of CHF. This, of course, made me smile again, because that's what I thought all along. The record was coded with accurate documentation and did not reflect conditions that were not present in this patient. Smile again; mission accomplished.

Lest you think all situations turn out with smiles, I have to tell you another story. Again this occurred in the ICU setting. I was reviewing a record when Dr. Explosive (again, the names have been changed to protect all parties, innocent or otherwise) was reviewing the record of his patient and was about 10–15 feet away from me. We were both quietly reviewing our records when Dr. Explosive started yelling in a loud and angry manner, "Who put this query here for me? Who is this 'Sheila Duhon?' This is a waste of my time! I will not be accosted like this when I am rounding!"

His meltdown caused all sorts of persons to stop doing whatever they were doing and all eyes were watching him. Patients' families came out of the rooms to see what all the ruckus was about. The nurse manager came flying from the other side of the unit to attempt damage control. Meanwhile, he kept ranting on and on, loudly and with great theatrics. I stood up and introduced myself and said I'd be happy to have a conversation with him about the query if he wanted to. He then proceeded to rip the query out of the chart (this was back in the days of paper charts) and threw the chart on the ground—papers (with all sorts of confidential information) strewn everywhere. He said he was not going to speak to me and stormed out of the ICU.

Ultimately, I brought my health information management (HIM) leadership into the loop. My supervisor, the ICU manager, and I proceeded to file an incident report of the event. The physician's behavior was addressed within a peer review process as well as from the hospital administrative team. And yes, the query did ultimately get answered. Deep breath and smile.

Let's talk about another scenario that essentially repeated itself over and over again with multiple physicians. Some physicians, when presented with a query, will just look at the CDI specialist and ask any number of the following questions:

- How do you want me to answer this?
- What do you want me to say?
- Just tell me what you want me to write.
- Can you write what you want and I'll just sign it?
- Which answer gets more money?

Now, I may be the only CDI specialist that has ever encountered this manner of response from a physician, but I doubt it. This seems to be a pretty common theme across our profession. So, what are we to do?

I finally learned how to get direct and to the point in my response to these questions. No amount of explaining my role, their independent clinical decision-making, their role as the attending physician, etc., ever seemed to make a difference. It still boiled down to the essence of "What do you want me to write?"

I changed my approach by simply redirecting that question right back in the form of "What I want you to write is *what, in your clinical judgment, is the condition you are treating. And then, describe that condition as specifically as you possibly can.*" This response seemed to ease tensions, as it is direct, to the point, and nonleading to be sure, but it also increased physician engagement. Smile and give yourself a pat on the back.

These personal examples are but a speck in the huge repertoire of CDI stories that can be recalled and shared with fellow CDI specialists. I share them not to imply that I have a magic potion that cures and removes all CDI obstacles, but rather to share that a sense of humor, a dedication to documentation of the truth and integrity of the medical record, and a bit of bravery when needed are all part of a day in the life of a CDI specialist.

The Physician Advisor

The role of the physician advisor is a relatively recent role, evolving from the need to more fully engage medical staff members and add credibility to CDI efforts. However, not all organizations incorporate the physician advisor model for CDI. Some lend support to the CDI program through the services of a physician champion, while others collaborate with the CDI initiative through the engagement of chief medical officers, medical department chairs, and medical chiefs of staff. These various roles with their corresponding titles collectively serve the CDI effort at the organization. The importance of having a well-respected and informed physician leader engage and understand the imperative nature of CDI is principal to the overall success of the CDI program irrespective of the title assigned.

Many organizations have established the physician leader role as a multidimensional role, incorporating responsibilities for case management, quality, coding, CDI, and other departments. Results from the 2017 CDI Week Industry Survey by ACDIS demonstrated the following in response to the question, "Does your department have a physician advisor or physician champion?"

PHYSICIAN ENGAGEMENT AND EDUCATION

Response	Response percent
Yes, we have a full-time physician advisor/champion	18.99%
Yes, we have a part-time physician advisor/champion	43.02%
No, but we plan on engaging one in the near future	12.85%
No, we have no plans to engage a physician advisor/champion	6.76%
Don't know	1.68%
Other (please specify)	6.70%

Source: 2017 CDI Week Industry Survey, ACDIS.

Additionally, the 2016 Physician Advisor Survey by ACDIS in partnership with Nuance demonstrated the following results regarding the distribution and sharing of the physician leader with other departments:

Department shared with	Shared %
Case Management	44%
Utilization Review	43%
Quality Department	21%
HIM & Coding	19%

Source: 2016 Physician Advisor Survey, ACDIS and Nuance.

Still other programs develop the physician advisor or physician leader role to act in silos, serving a singular department or program. The availability of physician advisors and leaders is in short supply across the nation, much like the shortage of CDI specialists. CDI programs committed to having an active and engaged physician advisor or leader enjoy the advantage of attracting medical staff engagement when one of their peers espouses and demonstrates the value and impact of this collaboration.

CHAPTER 2

The Physician Advisor's Role in CDI

There are several areas in which a physician advisor can be effective for both coding and CDI. Physician advisors are key in educating other physicians about the importance and impact of clear, precise, consistent, and reliable documentation. Connecting physician documentation to coding, which in turn drives publicly reported quality data, is just one aspect of the benefit of peer-to-peer physician education.

The physician advisor can relate the "collegial pain" of documenting for purposes beyond physician-to-physician communication. A physician advisor can explain that the medical record has evolved into a medical-legal record of enormous significance and lack of documentation specificity can be interpreted as substandard care rendered to the patient.

While the physician advisor is certainly a champion for CDI efforts, he or she is also an advocate for physicians, coding, the organization, and, ultimately, the patient. By acting as a mentor and educator to both physicians and CDI staff and coders, the chasm between clinical documentation language and coding language is narrowed. The CDI specialist is a liaison between the clinical world and the coding world. Much in the same way, the physician advisor is a liaison between the CDI specialist and the medical staff.

The physician advisor can also assist the CDI and coding staff with query compliance with a huge return on the investment of physician advisor time spent meeting with peers. Not every condition that lacks the utmost specificity and granularity in the code set necessitates a query. Coders are bound to follow the ICD-10-CM *Official Guidelines for Coding and Reporting*, which directs that codes can be submitted only for conditions that meet the following requirements:

- Clinical evaluation
- Therapeutic treatment
- Diagnostic procedures
- Extended length of hospital stay
- Increased nursing care and/or monitoring

Query compliance must follow these same guidelines. A query submitted for a condition that meets one or more of these requirements is appropriate. Conversely, a query submitted for incidental findings not meeting one or more of these requirements would be inappropriate. The physician advisor can often intervene and have a peer-to-peer conversation with physicians who do not respond to queries. This one-on-one communication often benefits all parties involved in support of the CDI program mission.

Personally, when I receive resistance to query responsiveness and comments to me, such as "You know this is acute systolic heart failure. Why are you asking me?" I often explain to physicians that I am not licensed to render diagnoses. I do not have the initials "MD" behind my name. However, the physician does have MD behind their name, and in the CDI world, *MD* means "*Make the Diagnosis.*" The physician is the final decision-maker and uses his or her independent clinical assessment regarding the diagnosis. Each physician has earned that exclusive prerogative, and only the physician can render a diagnosis.

The physician advisor must have excellent communication skills, be proficient at mentoring and educating peers, understand the business side of healthcare, and understand the impact documentation has on quality care delivery and scoring, utilization management, risk reduction for inaccurate coding and billing, and revenue performance. A capable physician advisor elicits support and cooperation from coding, CDI specialists, and physicians while facilitating a two-way communication channel between the parties.

A physician advisor can be a valuable asset to an organization in many ways. Few physician advisors are dedicated solely to CDI, as mentioned previously. Most are split between case management, CDI, and sometimes clinical quality as well. Therefore, use of the physician advisor's time is critically important and should be well planned. CDI specialists can and do perform a great deal of physician education in the world of documentation integrity. Nonetheless, when credentials behind the CDI specialist's name do not include MD, it's sometimes necessary and often extremely advantageous to bring the physician advisor into the conversation. The table below reflects the diversity of the physician advisor's scope of responsibilities, as respondents to the 2016 ACDIS Physician Advisor Survey reported.

CHAPTER 2

Physician advisor responsibilities	2016 Physician Advisor Survey	2016 Physician Advisor Survey for Physicians
Helping to "close" outstanding physician queries	58%	60%
Helping to draft compliant/effective queries	20%	42%
Querying physicians on a concurrent or retrospective basis	14%	26%
Offering coding/query suggestions to CDI/coding staff	33%	49%
Providing pre-/post-bill clinical documentation support	24%	42%
Assisting with auditor appeals/drafting appeals letters	37%	54%
Reviewing charts for medical necessity of inpatient admissions	30%	40%
Providing documentation/clinical education to CDI and coding staff	30%	47%
Assisting CDI staff with presenting documentation improvement education to physicians	55%	80%
Disciplining noncompliant physicians	34%	19%
Other	14%	10%

Source: 2016 Physician Advisor Survey, ACDIS and Nuance.

According to *The Physician Advisor's Guide to Clinical Documentation Improvement* by Trey La Charité, MD, FACP, SFHM, CCS, CCDS, and James S. Kennedy, MD, CCS, CDIP, effective physician advisors must possess a skill set that includes a high degree of credibility and respect with the medical staff at large. Expert communication skills, combined with a sound understanding of the revenue cycle and business aspect of the organization, is an additional foundation that empowers the physician leader to address with confidence and accuracy the principles that fellow physicians may not be aware of. A good working relationship with the organization's executive leadership team also goes a long way in understanding organizational needs and adapting to changing priorities that need communication to and buy-in from the medical staff.

One example of when the physician advisor/physician champion is invaluable is in the area of peer-to-peer communication, underscoring the relevance and impact of documentation integrity. This transcends gender, race, religion, nationality, and any other differences. Physicians respect other physicians and will listen to what their peers say. It's as simple as that. CDI specialists can benefit from that collegial relationship when in concert with the physician advisor. Ultimately, all parties benefit from the improved documentation; the patient's medical record is a document with the utmost integrity, and medical care rendered is memorialized in that record.

Speaking from a CDI specialist point of view, regardless of the exact title of the physician advisor, physician champion, physician consultant, or any other such designation, a physician who champions the cause of CDI is a strong ally that can propel the CDI specialists' efforts and the CDI program into an entirely different realm of effectiveness and impact. A CDI program that does not include a physician ally is likely not gleaning the best impact and value from the investment in the program and would be well advised to consider collaborating with a physician partner.

REFERENCES

The Association of Clinical Documentation Improvement Specialists & Nuance. (2016). *2016 Physician Advisor Survey* (Rep.). Middleton, MA: HCPro.

The Association of Clinical Documentation Improvement Specialists. (2017). *2017 CDI Week Industry Survey* (Rep.). Middleton, MA: HCPro.

The Association of Clinical Documentation Improvement Specialists. (2018). *2017 Salary Survey: Salaries continue to grow, but participants are less optimistic than in the past* (Rep.). Middleton, MA: HCPro.

Centers for Medicare and Medicaid Services, & National Center for Health Statistics. (2018). *ICD-10-CM Official Guidelines for Coding and Reporting.*

La Charité, T., & Kennedy, J. S. (2014). *The Physician Advisor's Guide to Clinical Documentation Improvement.* Middleton, MA: HCPro.

CHAPTER 3

A Compliant Query Practice

Historical Perspective

The query process was born from a need to glean specific clinical data and information that could be translated into alphanumeric codes. The alphanumeric codes were kept for statistical analysis to drive research and improved quality of medical care. In the United States, these codes were additionally used as the basis for payment to physicians and hospitals for the care and services rendered.

Queries were originally the domain of the professional coder and provided a mechanism to gain more specific documentation so more accurate code assignment could be delivered in the final legal and billable medical record. The query process was ill-defined and generally constructed by way of open-ended questions to the provider. Regulations surrounding legal and ethical ways to request additional documentation from providers were essentially nonexistent. Most organizations were left to internally define and self-regulate query compliance, a basis for potential misuse and abuse of the intent of query submission to code to the highest degree of specificity within the code set.

Clinical documentation improvement (CDI) programs began to appear in the 1990s in earnest, largely conceived as a means to close the gap between clinical and coding language and to streamline the coding, billing, and revenue cycle process. In essence, many programs were developed to improve financial processes associated with clinical record documentation.

The majority of the pioneer CDI specialists were recruited from the clinical world of registered nursing, according to the *2017 CDI Salary Survey* from the Association of Clinical Documentation Improvement Specialists (ACDIS). Nurses with a strong clinical foundation were trained in International

CHAPTER 3

Classification of Disease, Ninth Revision, Clinical Modification codes (abbreviated as ICD-9-CM; note that we have now moved to ICD-10-CM) and Diagnosis-Related Group (DRG) assignment. Emphasis on conditions that met the criteria for assignment as a complication or comorbid condition (CC) or as a major CC (MCC) were especially emphasized as needing specificity and documentation in the medical record. The Centers for Medicare & Medicaid Services (CMS) clearly stated that documentation requests for conditions that were monitored, evaluated, treated, or required additional length of hospital stay or nursing care were appropriate conditions to code and bill. This requirement holds true today as well.

With the introduction of clinically astute nurses into the clinical documentation process, a whole new set of issues arose. Certainly the benefit of a long-standing clinical relationship with the medical staff was realized; that was a win for both physicians and the health information management/coding (HIM) team. What was hard to reconcile was the nature and habits of nurses who had historically served as staunch patient advocates, ensuring the safest and best care was rendered to the patient at all times. This sometimes required some very direct communication on behalf of the patient. This direct style of communication was indeed often necessary and expected in the arena of clinical care. However, it did not serve the CDI programs well, most directly when it concerned query development. Queries developed by clinically trained nurses and physicians tended to be more direct, more leading, and therefore not aligned with coding guidelines. It became clear that more definitive guidance was necessary surrounding query development.

Authoritative Guidance

AHIMA

The American Health Information Management Association (AHIMA) has published several successive practice briefs to address the topics of developing and managing effective and compliant query processes and CDI programs:

- 2001: *Developing a Physician Query Process*
- 2008: *Managing an Effective Query Process*
- 2010: *Guidance for Clinical Documentation Improvement Programs*
- 2011: *AHIMA Code of Ethics*

A COMPLIANT QUERY PRACTICE

- 2013: *Guidelines for Achieving a Compliant Query Practice* (now retired)
- 2016: *Ethical Standards for Clinical Documentation Improvement Professionals*
- 2016: *Guidelines for Achieving a Compliant Query Practice*, updated from 2013 and coauthored with ACDIS
- 2016: *Clinical Documentation Improvement Toolkit*
- 2016: *Clinical Validation: The Next Level of CDI*

ACDIS

Over the years, as the CDI profession has grown, ACDIS has gained prominence as the leading organization dedicated solely to the growing CDI profession. ACDIS has published several white papers and position papers since its inception in 2007 on a wide array of topics addressing key topics in the CDI profession:

- 2013: *Electronic health records and the role of the CDI specialist*
- 2014: *Defining the CDI specialist's roles and responsibilities*
- 2015: *ACDIS Code of Ethics*
- 2015: *Cornerstone of CDI success: Build a strong foundation*
- 2015: *Ten things you need to know about ICD-10—and tell your physicians*
- 2015: *Physician queries and the use of prior information: Reevaluating the role of the CDI specialist*
- 2015: *Post-acute CDI: An introduction to long-term acute care hospitals*
- 2016: *New definitions of sepsis and septic shock: Response from the ACDIS Advisory Board*
- 2016: *Guidelines for Achieving a Compliant Query Practice*, updated from 2013 and coauthored with AHIMA
- 2016: *Outpatient clinical documentation improvement: An introduction*
- 2016: *From finance to quality: CDI departments expanding their reach*
- 2016: *Pediatric respiratory failure: The need for specific definitions*
- 2016: *Keep staff growing and engaged with a CDI career ladder*

CHAPTER 3

- 2016: *Set CDI productivity expectations, but don't look for a national standard*
- 2017: *CDI: More than a credential*
- 2017: *Where are we now with sepsis?*
- 2017: *Clinical validation and the role of the CDI professional*
- 2017: *CDI and the evolution from finance to quality*
- 2017: *Developing effective CDI leadership: A matter of effort and attitude*
- 2018: *Queries in outpatient CDI: Developing a compliant, effective process*
- 2018: *The pros and cons of remote CDI: Evaluate before you implement*
- 2018: *Find the right vendor for your organization: Best practice for getting started*
- 2018: *Coding an acute myocardial infarction: Unraveling the mystery*

The Health Insurance Portability and Accountability Act (HIPAA) and the four Cooperating Parties

The Health Insurance Portability and Accountability Act (HIPAA) enacted in 1996 mandated adherence to the *Reporting and Coding Guidelines*, derived from the four agencies who oversee the development of these guidelines annually. These agencies are collectively known as the "Cooperating Parties" and consist of the following organizations:

- AHIMA
- CMS
- American Hospital Association (AHA)
- National Center for Health Statistics (NCHS)

AHIMA advises that healthcare entities should develop policies and procedures that clarify which clinical conditions and documentation situations warrant a request for physician clarification. Compliance oversight programs are integral to ensuring queries are presented for appropriate conditions, in a nonleading manner, and meet legal and ethical standards. A CDI program that aligns itself in partnership with a compliance program is likely to remain above reproach for unethical or illegal practices.

The False Claims Act and the Stark Law

A compliant query program and process that self-monitors, audits, educates, and corrects inaccurate code assignment and billing when discovered. Laws intended to discourage false claims and billing include the following:

- The False Claims Act is a federal law that makes it a crime for any person or organization to knowingly make a false record or file a false claim regarding any federal healthcare program, which includes any plan or program that provides health benefits, whether directly, through insurance or otherwise, which is funded directly, in whole or in part, by the United States Government or any state healthcare system. In summation, the False Claims Act imposes liability on any person who submits a claim to the federal government that he or she knows (or should know) is false.

    – An interesting fact about the False Claims Act is that it is also referred to as the "Lincoln Law," as it was signed into law on March 2, 1862, by President Abraham Lincoln to discourage false billing to the federal government during the United States Civil War. The law underwent numerous changes in 1986 and significantly increased damages levied against persons found guilty. The United States Department of Justice and the Office of Inspector General investigate and bring suit against healthcare individuals and organizations that disobey the law.

- The Stark Law is a section of the Social Security Act that addresses physician self-referral. The Stark Law prohibits a physician from making referrals for certain designated health services (DHS) payable by Medicare to any entity in which there exists a financial relationship that will benefit the physician.

The existence of such laws points to the very serious nature of filing and billing claims for medical care. The consequences of violations include financial penalties and/or incarceration.

Practicing physicians understand the legalities of false claims and may associate the query process as an attempt by an organization or individual to increase revenue or data scoring. Physicians must understand legal billing and claim submissions as a matter of fulfilling the contractual agreement with CMS and other payers. It is not uncommon to hear a physician refer to his or her office manager as the person he or she relies on most heavily to keep the office billing within legal and compliant coding and billing practices. In the hospital setting, it is equally vital to establish and follow a compliant query process. The HIM and

CHAPTER 3

CDI programs must comply with legal and ethical standards set by the federal government, CMS, and the Cooperating Parties.

The Query Process

AHIMA and ACDIS joint brief, 2016

The joint brief, updated in 2016, on a compliant query practice from AHIMA and ACDIS defines a query as:

> *A communication tool used to clarify documentation in the health record for accurate code assignment. The desired outcome from a query is an update of a health record to better reflect a practitioner's intent and clinical thought processes, documented in a manner that supports accurate code assignment. All professionals are encouraged to adhere to these compliant querying guidelines regardless of credential, role, title, or use of any technological tools involved in the query process.*

The joint brief further states that, "In court, an attorney can't 'lead' a witness into a statement. In hospitals, coders and clinical documentation specialists can't lead healthcare providers with queries. Therefore, appropriate etiquette must be followed when querying providers for additional health record information."

The AHIMA 6

In the practice brief, ACDIS and AHIMA clearly define the circumstances under which a query is appropriate. More commonly known as the "AHIMA 6," the following circumstances direct when a query to the physician is warranted and ethical.

- When documentation is **illegible**: Illegibility is generally defined as when three or more clinical experts cannot decipher the handwritten documentation. In the world of ever-increasing electronic medical record documentation, this is becoming less common as a circumstance to query.

- When documentation is **incomplete**: Incomplete documentation may occur when treatment is rendered and/or test results indicate a diagnosis that has not been fully documented by the physician.

- When documentation is **ambiguous**: Ambiguous documentation may be present when signs and symptoms are present, tested, and/or treated, but no clear statement of etiology is documented by the provider.

- When documentation is **inconsistent**: Inconsistent documentation may present in the form of a

A COMPLIANT QUERY PRACTICE

diagnosis or condition appearing in the medical record on a sporadic basis, not followed through daily until the condition is resolved. It may also present as documentation that flips back and forth between two or more conditions as if the conditions are the same and interchangeable.

- When documentation is **imprecise**: Imprecise documentation presents as an opportunity for greater specificity or granularity of the condition as supported by clinical indicators such as test results, physical exam findings, and response to interventions, treatments, and medications.

- When documentation is **conflicting or unreliable**: Conflicting documentation among providers requires further clarification in the form of a query. CMS assigns the attending physician as the physician of record with the final responsibility to assign diagnoses, thus superseding all other providers of care.

Some additional scenarios that may require clarification in the form of a query are:

- The presence of clinical indicators or data without a corresponding diagnosis
- The presence of clinical indicators that suggest a higher degree of specificity of a condition is likely
- To establish or rule out a cause and effect relationship between conditions and/or organisms
- Signs and symptoms without a documented etiology or associated condition
- Clarification of the onset of a condition, most notably when determining whether a condition is present on admission (POA)

What is a leading query?

"A leading query is one that is not supported by the clinical elements in the health record and/or directs a provider to a specific diagnosis or procedure," according to the ACDIS/AHIMA practice brief. Any diagnosis that is obtained through a leading query must be removed from the final coded record. Additionally, steps should be taken to educate the query author and a process initiated to audit the performance and demonstrated improvement by the query author.

A leading query might be a query that offers the provider only higher-weighted (and therefore higher-reimbursement) options for response. It might also be a query that consists of clinical indicators that are "edited" by the query author to include only those that would lead to a specific diagnosis. If the question posed to the physician includes a supposed or desired diagnosis, then the query might risk being leading, especially when asked in a yes/no format. "Although open-ended queries are preferred, multiple choice and 'yes/no'

CHAPTER 3

queries are also acceptable under certain circumstances," according to the practice brief. CDI specialists are well advised to study the guidelines and position papers from ACDIS and AHIMA carefully to ensure query development that is appropriate and compliant while reducing risk for denial and assertions of fraud.

Below is an example of a leading query from the ACDIS/AHIMA joint query practice brief.

Noncompliant query example

Clinical scenario:

On admission, bilateral lower extremity edema is noted, however, there are no other clinical indicators to support malnutrition.

Query:

Do you agree that the patient's bilateral lower extremity edema is diagnostic of malnutrition? Please document your response in the health record or below.

- Yes _____
- No _____
- Other _____
- Clinically Undetermined _____

Name: _____ Date: _____

Rationale:

Malnutrition is not a further specification of the isolated finding of a bilateral lower extremity edema. An open-ended or multiple-choice query should be used under this circumstance to ascertain the underlying cause of the patient's edema.

Source: This sample query was taken from the joint ACDIS/AHIMA publication, "Guidelines for Achieving a Compliant Query Practice," which was updated in 2016.

What is a compliant query?

The components of a compliant query include:

- **Demographic data**: Information including patient and encounter identifiers, date, physician information, and other key data elements.

A COMPLIANT QUERY PRACTICE

- **Clinical indicators**: Patient-specific clinical information that directly correlates to the focus and intent of the query submission. According to the ACDIS/AHIMA Practice Brief, "Clinical indicators should be derived from the specific medical record under review and the unique episode of care. Clinical indicators supporting the query may include elements from the entire medical record, such as diagnostic findings and provider impressions."

- **Question or request**: A nonleading request for clarification of a condition or documentation in the record that requires further specificity to accurately code, resulting in accurate reflection of the severity of illness, risk of mortality, and intensity of services provided to treat the condition.

- **Provider response**: The physician's response to a query should be well defined by organization policy and procedure. The response should be "memorialized" in either a written format or the electronic medical record.

Query Storage and Retrieval

Queries may be kept as a component of the legal medical record or may be separate from the legal medical record. The governing bodies do not mandate that the query be retained as a component of the legal medical record, but ACDIS and AHIMA do recommend that organizations that do not include the query in the legal medical record develop and maintain a system for retaining the queries a part of the business record.

Retrieval of the query and the response may be necessary for future legal, ethical, or compliance inquiries regarding the medical record and documentation. When the organization requires or provides the option for the provider to respond to the query on the query form itself, it should always be maintained as a permanent part of the legal medical record.

The verbal query versus the written query

A query may be posed to the physician either in a written or a verbal format. Irrespective of the format, however, the same guidelines apply. A verbal query cannot lead a physician to a specific response. Neither can the effect on physician or hospital profile scoring be indicated. No discussion of reimbursement is allowed. At all times, the clinical indicators discussed must pertain to the focus of the query and allow the physician to exercise his or her own independent clinical judgment in providing a response. Verbal queries should be "memorialized" in writing at the time of the query discussion or very soon thereafter.

CHAPTER 3

In some instances, a verbal query may be preferable to a written one. The opportunity to have a face-to-face discussion with the physician is a natural lead in to the verbal query approach. This scenario often presents itself when the CDI specialist is on-site at the point of care or when telephone communication is optimized for the CDI process. When talking with the provider, the relevant clinical indicators that demonstrate the need for greater specificity in the record should be discussed, and the possible options for response are still within the same boundaries as would be present in the written query format.

According to the ACDIS/AHIMA practice brief, "Because the patient record should provide a sequence of events, best practice is to capture the content of a verbal and/or written query, as well as any practitioner response to the query. This practice allows reviewers to account for the presence [of] documentation that might otherwise appear out of context." Just as importantly, the brief continues to say that, "The justification (i.e., inclusion of relevant clinical indicators) for the query is more important than the query format." Therefore, whether you're using a verbal or a written approach, the best practice is to always adhere closely to compliant query guidelines.

There Is No Correct or Incorrect Response to a Query

It is important to make a point to the physician that there is no right or wrong answer for any query. At times a physician may truly not be certain or comfortable enough to diagnose a condition with greater specificity. A response of "unable to determine" or "unknown" is an acceptable response, and CDI specialists should be willing to accept this type of response.

When physicians understand that the intent of the query is simply to obtain the greatest specificity possible—it is not an indictment or judgment of the care the physician is providing—we are likely to gain more acceptance and cooperation with the query process. It is important to clearly communicate to the physician that greater specificity in the medical record more accurately reflects the true complexity of the care they are providing and the extent of the medical decision-making involved. The CDI specialist is uniquely poised to assist the physician in ensuring that the medical record reflects the true complexity of medical skills and knowledge the physician possesses.

The Concurrent Query Process

CDI specialists most often submit queries concurrently, while the patient is still in the hospital or undergoing treatment. Concurrent queries provide timely clarification, reflective of the true severity of illness, risk of mortality, and intensity of services required to care for the patient. This real-time accurate documentation drives the concurrent coding and DRG assignment. This is valuable information to many stakeholders: the physicians providing care have more complete and precise documentation with which they communicate to each other, the case management team has a more precise length of stay estimates to assist in discharge planning, the business office has more accurate forecasting data to determine resource allocation, and the quality department has real-time actionable data to drive improved outcomes for patients.

The Retrospective Query Process

Retrospective queries are initiated after the patient is discharged from the facility. A retrospective query may be initiated by the coding professional when documentation is such that the record cannot be accurately coded and sent for billing until the incomplete, imprecise, ambiguous, inconsistent, illegible, or unreliable documentation is addressed.

Traditionally, the retrospective query is within the scope of the coding professional; however, on occasion, a CDI specialist may submit a retrospective query. This often occurs when the CDI specialist is tasked with performing retrospective reviews as part of risk reduction efforts for denials, review of the accuracy of codes that feed to public data, and other such organization-specific initiatives.

When CDI specialists engage in retrospective reviews and queries, it's critical to maintain awareness of the risk for what I call "CDI scope creep." The temptation to review the record for more than documentation incongruences may result in expectations for CDI professionals that step outside the boundaries of the official coding and reporting guidelines as determined by the Cooperating Parties. By this I mean that CDI professionals should be very cautious when performing retrospective reviews that may accompany expectations that the retrospective review will drive more favorable data reporting.

Note the caution from the AHIMA Standards of Ethical Coding (2016 version): "Coding professionals **shall not:** Misrepresent the patient's clinical picture through intentional incorrect coding or omission of diagnosis or procedure codes, or the addition of diagnosis or procedure codes unsupported by health record documentation, to inappropriately increase reimbursement, justify medical necessity, improve publicly reported data, or qualify for insurance policy coverage benefits." The expectations for retrospective queries are the same as for concurrent queries: each must adhere to the "AHIMA 6" criteria for compliant queries.

When a Provider Refuses to Respond to a Query

In the perfect CDI world, all queries posed to providers would be answered in a timely manner. But, we all know that, sometimes, this is not the case. When the CDI specialist has performed due diligence in query development, and appropriate communication of the query has been presented to the physician, it may be proper to enlist the assistance of the physician advisor (or physician designee/champion). Ultimately, support of the query process ensures the integrity of the documentation and final coding. Active support and engagement from the C-suite and medical staff leadership are invaluable in determining the impact the CDI program will demonstrate for the organization.

According to the ACDIS/AHIMA practice brief:

> CMS recommends that each facility develop an escalation policy for unanswered queries and to address any staff concerns regarding queries. In the event that a query does not receive a professional response, the case should be referred for further review in accordance with the facility's escalation policy. The escalation process may include, but is not limited to, referral to a physician advisor, the chief medical officer, or other administrative personnel.

Authorized Persons Who Can Query a Provider

The responsibility for query submission lies within the scope of a specially trained/certified professional coder or a CDI specialist. Queries are not within the scope of practice for others in such fields as case management, quality, business office, or revenue cycle. According to the AHIMA *Standards of Ethical Coding*, the standards are intended,

> To assist and guide coding professionals whether credentialed or not; including but not limited to coding staff, coding auditors, coding educators, clinical documentation improvement (CDI) professionals, and managers responsible for decision-making processes and operations as well as HIM/coding students. The standards outline expectations for making ethical decisions in the workplace and demonstrate coding professionals' commitment to integrity during the coding process, regardless of the purpose for which the codes are being reported.

A COMPLIANT QUERY PRACTICE

Coding professionals and CDI specialists are further guided in the *Standards of Ethical Coding* to "Refuse to participate in and/or conceal unethical coding, data abstraction, query practices, or any inappropriate activities related to coding and address any perceived unethical coding-related practices."

The Query Format

Query style or format is not mandated by query guidelines. Some organizations may choose to develop queries as open-ended and freestyle, while other organizations may develop templates designed to ensure query guideline compliance by each individual query author. Whichever approach is adopted, a regular audit and review process is recommended to ensure the queries issued are consistently compliant. Compliance auditors knowledgeable in coding and query guidance should audit and make recommendations for education and process changes as necessary. Audits may be performed internally or by an external auditing company. Regardless of the route chosen, it is imperative that audit results are taken seriously, with definitive steps taken to correct deficiencies identified.

Queries can be posed to physicians in open-ended, multiple-choice, or yes/no formats. Let's look at each one.

Open-ended queries

- Should include an open-ended, nonleading question or request for clarification that allows a freestyle response from the physician

CHAPTER 3

> **Open-ended query example**
>
> **Clinical scenario:**
>
> A patient is admitted with pneumonia. The admitting H&P examination reveals WBC of 14,000, a respiratory rate of 24, a temperature of 102 degrees, heart rate of 120, hypotension, and altered mental status. The patient is administered an IV antibiotic and IV fluid resuscitation.
>
> **Query:**
>
> Based on your clinical judgment, can you provide a diagnosis that represents the below-listed clinical indicators?
>
> In this patient admitted with pneumonia, the admitting history and physical examination reveals the following:
>
> - WBC, 14,000
> - Respiratory rate, 24
> - Temperature, 102°F
> - Heart rate, 120
> - Hypotension
> - Altered mental status
> - IV antibiotic administration
> - IV fluid resuscitation
>
> Please document the condition and the causative organism (if known) in the medical record.

Source: This sample query was taken from the joint ACDIS/AHIMA publication, "Guidelines for Achieving a Compliant Query Practice," which was updated in 2016.

Multiple-choice queries

- Should include clinically significant and reasonable options as supported by clinical indicators in the record

- Providing a new diagnosis as an option in a multiple-choice list (as supported and substantiated by referenced clinical indicators from the health record) is not introducing new information and is therefore allowed

- Should include both higher-weighted and lower-weighted options for response

- Should include "other" and "unable to determine/unknown" as options for response

A COMPLIANT QUERY PRACTICE

> **Multiple-choice query example**
>
> **Clinical scenario:**
>
> A patient is admitted for a right hip fracture. The H&P notes that the patient has a history of chronic congestive heart failure. A recent echocardiogram showed left ventricular ejection fraction (EF) of 25%. The patient's home medications include metoprolol XL, lisinopril, and Lasix.
>
> **Query:**
>
> It is noted in the impression of the H&P that the patient has chronic congestive heart failure and a recent echocardiogram noted under the cardiac review of systems reveals an EF of 25%. Can the chronic heart failure be further specified as:
>
> - Chronic systolic heart failure _____
> - Chronic diastolic heart failure _____
> - Chronic systolic and diastolic heart failure _____
> - Some other type of heart failure _____
> - Undetermined _____

Source: This sample query was taken from the joint ACDIS/AHIMA publication, "Guidelines for Achieving a Compliant Query Practice," which was updated in 2016.

Yes/no queries

- Must include the options yes, no, other, and clinically undetermined, or unknown
- Do not use yes/no queries where only clinical indicators of a condition are present, but the specific condition/diagnosis has not been documented in the record
- A new diagnosis cannot be introduced by a yes/no query

CHAPTER 3

> **Yes/no query example**
>
> **Clinical scenario:**
>
> A patient is admitted with cellulitis around a recent operative wound site, and only cellulitis is documented without any relationship to the recent surgical procedure.
>
> **Query:**
>
> Is the cellulitis due to or the result of the surgical procedure? Please document your response in the health record or below.
>
> - Yes _____
> - No _____
> - Other _____
> - Clinically undetermined _____

Source: This sample query was taken from the joint ACDIS/AHIMA publication, "Guidelines for Achieving a Compliant Query Practice," which was updated in 2016.

Writing Effective Queries: Best Practices

Writing effective, compliant queries takes practice, a sound clinical foundation, an understanding of the physician mindset and perspective, a thorough understanding of coding guidelines, and lots of patience! In the following section, we will explore tips and techniques that may help you master this vital element of the CDI process.

The "TRIC" to query success

The **TRIC** approach to queries provides a quick and systematic approach that ensures the necessary components of the query are present and displayed in a compliant manner to the provider. **TRIC** is the acronym that stands for these four components: treatment, risk, indicators, and compliant question.

1. **T**reatment: Coding guidelines mandate that any condition coded and reported must be relevant to the encounter for care (see the 2018 *Official Guidelines for Coding and Reporting*). A condition must be monitored, treated, and evaluated, require increased allocation of nursing resources, or require an extended stay. Therefore, when a query is posed to the provider, there should exist and be

documented in the query clear and precise indicators of treatment, monitoring, evaluation, increased allocation of nursing resources, or extended-stay requirements. Findings that are incidental and insignificant are not considered relevant to the encounter and should not be used as documentation in a query. Additionally, such findings should not be coded.

2. **R**isk: Risk refers to the relevance of the diagnosis to the patient and the encounter for care. Signs and symptoms can be brought into account when assessing risk. For example, a diagnosis of pneumonia in an elderly bed-bound patient with a history of a cerebrovascular accident and a diagnosis of dysphagia with an impaired gag reflex possesses a risk for the more complex diagnosis of aspiration pneumonia.

3. **I**ndicators: Indicators refer to the clinical indicators that comprise the overall clinical picture inclusive of the risk, treatment, response to intervention, and test findings that are taken into account during the physician's medical decision-making process and assessment to arrive at a diagnosis. A query should contain sufficient clinical indicators that would support (or rule out) a diagnosis. Therefore, presenting a single clinical indicator, such as an abnormal laboratory test finding without corresponding signs, symptoms, treatment, or response to treatment, would likely render a query noncompliant and perhaps leading in nature.

4. **C**ompliant question: The compliant question should always be clear and succinct. Always be professional, courteous, and include your contact information so that the physician may contact you for any questions he or she may have about the query or other documentation issues. If a physician responds to a query by countering and asking what you're asking, you may not have stated your question clearly and succinctly. If the question was clear and succinct, then study the other components of the query. Were the clinical indicators aligned with the condition(s) of the query focus? Was there risk to the patient associated with the focus of the query? Was there correlation of treatments and interventions to the condition? If you can answer in the negative to any of these questions, you may want to analyze the query components and practice more effective query writing.

Chapter 4 in this book contains scenarios that will assist you in learning how to more effectively identify query opportunities, tie in all the TRIC components of a query, and more effectively construct compliant and impactful queries.

CHAPTER 3

The "dos" for an effective query process

If you incorporate these practices and tenets into your query development, you will find your queries are clearer, more direct in intent (but not directing in terms of response desired from the provider), and to the point, with results more aligned with the CDI process.

All queries should include the following items:

- Clinical indicators in a bullet-point or numbered format in a concise and precise manner (long paragraphs and sentences are generally not concise and precise and therefore should be avoided whenever possible)
- Patient-specific clinical indicators that are relevant to the question
- Citations regarding where the clinical indicator is located in the medical record
- Citations regarding who documented the clinical indicator in the medical record
- Citations regarding when the clinical indicator was documented in the medical record

CDI specialists should always proofread the query prior to submission to check for spelling, grammatical, and formatting errors. Queries are submitted to highly educated professionals who are typically short on time. Therefore, do your best to eliminate time-wasting components of a query that are not relevant to the intent of the query. Avoid losing credibility with the physician by presenting queries that are easy to decipher, are well written and without grammatical, spelling, or formatting errors, and are direct and to the point. Such efforts on the part of the CDI professional are generally better received and therefore stand a better chance of engagement and response from the provider. In short, if you are going to take the time and effort to submit a query, do it right—each and every time.

The "don'ts" for an effective query process

If you avoid the following pitfalls, your query results will be more meaningful and useful for data collection. Additionally, the query will effectively ensure that the record accurately reflects the patient's true medical conditions.

Compliant queries should never:

- Indicate the impact on reimbursement, DRG, length of stay, or relative weight
- Indicate the impact on physician or organization quality scoring or profiling
- Indicate the impact or addition of a CC or MCC
- Paraphrase or summarize findings in your own words

Developing an effective, compliant, and impactful query process takes time, education, and practice. A new CDI specialist will likely work closely with an experienced CDI specialist or coding professional to learn and hone the skills necessary to develop "submission-worthy" queries. Adding this skill to the repertoire of skills necessary for the CDI specialist requires a learning curve—sometimes a steep one! Developing clinically sound, coding-compliant query skills, however, is immeasurable in terms of impact and value added to the organization's CDI mission.

REFERENCES

The American Health Information Management Association. (2011). *AHIMA Code of Ethics* (Rep.). Chicago, IL: AHIMA.

The American Health Information Management Association. (2016). *Clinical Documentation Improvement Toolkit* (Rep.). Chicago, IL: AHIMA.

The American Health Information Management Association. (2016). *Clinical Validation: The Next Level of CDI* (Rep.). Chicago, IL: AHIMA.

The American Health Information Management Association. (2001). *Developing a Physician Query Process* (Rep.). Chicago, IL: AHIMA.

The American Health Information Management Association. (2016). *Ethical Standards for Clinical Documentation Improvement Professionals* (Rep.). Chicago, IL: AHIMA.

The American Health Information Management Association. (2010). *Guidance for Clinical Documentation Improvement Programs* (Rep.). Chicago, IL: AHIMA.

The American Health Information Management Association. (2013). *Guidelines for Achieving a Compliant Query Practice* (Rep.). Chicago, IL: AHIMA.

The American Health Information Management Association. (2008). *Managing an Effective Query Process* (Rep.). Chicago, IL: AHIMA.

The American Health Information Management Association, & The Association of Clinical Documentation Improvement Specialists. (2016). *Guidelines for Achieving a Compliant Query Practice* (Rep.). Chicago, IL: AHIMA.

The Association of Clinical Documentation Improvement Specialists. (2018). *2017 Salary Survey: Salaries continue to grow, but participants are less optimistic than in the past* (Rep.). Middleton, MA: HCPro.

CHAPTER 3

The Association of Clinical Documentation Improvement Specialists. (2015). *ACDIS Code of Ethics* (Rep.). Middleton, MA: HCPro.

The Association of Clinical Documentation Improvement Specialists. (2017). *CDI: More Than a Credential* (Rep.). Middleton, MA: HCPro.

The Association of Clinical Documentation Improvement Specialists. (2017). *Clinical Validation and the Role of the CDI Professional* (Rep.). Middleton, MA: HCPro.

The Association of Clinical Documentation Improvement Specialists. (2015). *Cornerstone of CDI Success: Build a Strong Foundation* (Rep.). Middleton, MA: HCPro.

The Association of Clinical Documentation Improvement Specialists. (2014). *Defining the CDI Specialist's Roles and Responsibilities* (Rep.). Middleton, MA: HCPro.

The Association of Clinical Documentation Improvement Specialists. (2017). *Developing Effective CDI Leadership: A Matter of Effort and Attitude* (Rep.). Middleton, MA: HCPro.

The Association of Clinical Documentation Improvement Specialists. (2013). *Electronic Health Records and the Role of the CDI Specialist* (Rep.). Middleton, MA: HCPro.

The Association of Clinical Documentation Improvement Specialists. (2018). *Find the Right Vendor for Your Organization: Best Practice for Getting Started* (Rep.). Middleton, MA: HCPro.

The Association of Clinical Documentation Improvement Specialists. (2016). *From Finance to Quality: CDI Departments Expanding Their Reach* (Rep.). Middleton, MA: HCPro.

The Association of Clinical Documentation Improvement Specialists. (2016). *New Definitions of Sepsis and Septic Shock: Response from the ACDIS Advisory Board* (Rep.). Middleton, MA: HCPro.

The Association of Clinical Documentation Improvement Specialists. (2016). *Outpatient Clinical Documentation Improvement: An Introduction* (Rep.). Middleton, MA: HCPro.

The Association of Clinical Documentation Improvement Specialists. (2016). *Pediatric Respiratory Failure: The Need for Specific Definitions* (Rep.). Middleton, MA: HCPro.

The Association of Clinical Documentation Improvement Specialists. (2015). *Physician Queries and the Use of Prior Information: Reevaluating the Role of the CDI Specialist* (Rep.). Middleton, MA: HCPro.

The Association of Clinical Documentation Improvement Specialists. (2015). *Postacute CDI: An Introduction to Long-Term Acute Care Hospitals* (Rep.). Middleton, MA: HCPro.

The Association of Clinical Documentation Improvement Specialists. (2018). *The Pros and Cons of Remote CDI: Evaluate Before You Implement* (Rep.). Middleton, MA: HCPro.

The Association of Clinical Documentation Improvement Specialists. (2018). *Queries in Outpatient CDI: Developing a Compliant, Effective Process* (Rep.). Middleton, MA: HCPro.

The Association of Clinical Documentation Improvement Specialists. (2016). *Set CDI Productivity Expectations, But Don't Look for a National Standard* (Rep.). Middleton, MA: HCPro.

The Association of Clinical Documentation Improvement Specialists. (2015). *Ten Things You Need to Know About ICD-10—And Tell Your Physicians* (Rep.). Middleton, MA: HCPro.

The Association of Clinical Documentation Improvement Specialists. (2017). *Where Are We Now with Sepsis?* (Rep.). Middleton, MA: HCPro.

CHAPTER 4

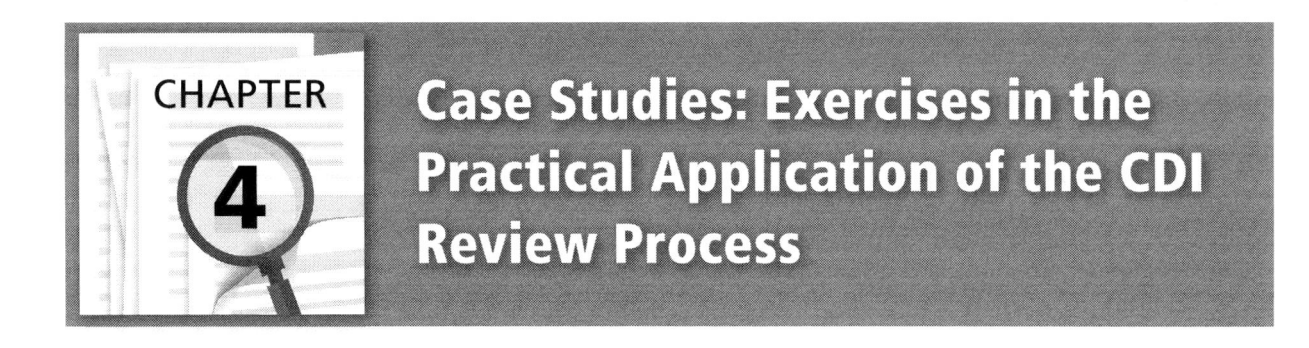

Case Studies: Exercises in the Practical Application of the CDI Review Process

Tips for Reviewing the Case Studies

The content contained in this chapter will undoubtedly present opportunities for lively and passionate discussions, sometimes debates, and at other times outright disagreement among clinical documentation improvement (CDI) specialists. It is my hope that it will also give you greater insight and reassurance that all is not "black or white" in the CDI query process; rather, there are several shades of gray, and navigating through them often requires a critical analysis of the entire clinical scenario.

A keen understanding of coding guidelines will also serve the CDI specialist well. Partnership with coding professionals is an invaluable asset to have in the CDI toolkit: I am certain my foundation in the CDI world is solidly grounded in coding fundamentals taught to me by my coding manger. I am grateful for her guidance and patience as she taught me the "coding language" that is foreign to most clinical professionals. So, take heed and learn from your coding teammates! They are wise to learn the "clinical language" from you as well. It truly takes the best from each of us to achieve excellence from all.

This is the world the CDI specialist lives in daily when faced with documentation that may need further clarification by the provider. We often ask ourselves such questions as:

- Is this documentation unclear? Imprecise? Inconsistent? Illegible? Incomplete? Unreliable? And, if so, is this condition relevant to the current encounter for care?

- Is it too early to query? Or should I wait another day?

- Will the physician be irritated with me if I query for this specificity?

- If I don't pose this query, will that negatively affect the data that my leadership reviews to assess my competency and impact?

- Will this query make a difference in the final Diagnosis-Related Group (DRG) assignment?

- Will the response affect the final severity of illness (SOI) or risk of mortality (ROM)?

- Will this query delay the final coding and negatively impact the business operations and revenue cycle of the organization?

- How can I pose this query in a compliant and nonleading manner?

- I already have several complications or comorbid conditions (CC) or major CCs (MCC) in the record; should I really pose a query that will result in yet another CC or MCC?

If only the answers to these questions—swirling around and around in every CDI specialist's brain daily—were so simple. Yet, in some ways, we can simplify it. The real question comes down to the integrity of the medical record. If the condition is relevant to the encounter and can be further specified, then yes, the CDI specialist should likely query for that additional specificity to more accurately reflect the patient's clinical condition. The number of preceding CCs or MCCs, the change (or no change) in the DRG, and all these other questions are not germane to the mission of CDI: to ensure that the final medical record is the truest reflection of the patient's clinical scenario. CDI is not about getting more CCs or MCCs. It is not about "maximizing" the DRG or the SOI/ROM scores. It is not about making the geometric length of stay (GMLOS) fit the actual length of stay (LOS), nor is it about ensuring quality data reflects reporting of superior public data. Clinical documentation integrity is just that: integrity. The truth of the clinical condition—that is the true mission of CDI.

As you work through the clinical scenarios in this chapter, I encourage you to work alone, work in teams, and use the case studies as a forum for discussion among coding professionals and CDI specialists. Take notes as you read through the case studies—we've left you space for that. The formatting of the case study presentations in this workbook is intentionally designed to be used as an ongoing exercise. Employ the scenarios to engage with and as a prelude to discussions with your physicians.

In short, use these scenarios and the points of discussion and education within each to build robust and challenging conversations that drive each of us to a higher level of performance and impact within the CDI profession.

CASE STUDIES: EXERCISES IN THE PRACTICAL APPLICATION OF THE CDI REVIEW PROCESS

Case Study: Neurology

Altered mental status

Physician documentation

History of present illness: The patient is an 88-year-old female who denies any past medical history but is significantly confused at the present time. She is oriented to self only; baseline mental status is unknown. She was brought to the emergency department (ED) by a neighbor and the family cannot be contacted at this time. She is admitted with altered mental status (AMS) most likely secondary to electrolyte imbalance and dehydration.

Past medical history: Unable to ascertain at this time. The patient is not a reliable historian and no family is present. The neighbor states that the patient has diabetes (DM) but is unsure if the patient takes medication for her diabetes.

Home medications: Unknown at this time.

Physical exam:

- Heart: Regular rate and rhythm
- Lungs: Clear to auscultation
- Mentation: Confused, cooperative, Glasgow Coma Scale (GCS) score 14
- Integumentary: Skin is warm, dry, poor skin turgor and + tenting bilateral hands
- Vital signs: blood pressure (BP) 114/52; heart rate (HR) 76; respiratory rate (RR) 16; temperature 99.0°F; O_2 saturation 96% on room air (RA)

Treatment: Careful hydration with IV fluids, normal saline 0.9% at 125 ml/hour. Neuro checks q two hours, contact family for patient history and discharge planning.

Clinical findings

Radiology: Computed tomography (CT) of the brain report—No evidence of acute intracranial abnormalities. Diffuse microvascular chronic changes noted.

LABORATORY RESULTS

	Day 3	Day 2	Day 1
Na+	136	131 (L)	128 (L)
K+	4.5	4.9	5.6 (H)
Blood glucose	118 (H)	126 (H)	278 (H)
BUN	13	23 (H)	30 (H)
Creatinine	0.78	1.06 (H)	1.35 (H)
GFR	>60.0	49.6 (L)	37.5 (L)
Drug screen			Negative
ETOH screen			Negative
UA—leukocyte esterase			Negative
UA—nitrite			Negative
UA—specific gravity			1.052 (H)
UA—glucose (mg/dl)			>1000 (H)
Hgb A1c			13.2 (H)

CASE STUDIES: EXERCISES IN THE PRACTICAL APPLICATION OF THE CDI REVIEW PROCESS

GLASGOW COMA SCALE

	GCS Score	Day 2 Score	Day 1 Score
Eye opening			
• Spontaneous	4		4
• Response to verbal command	3		
• Response to pain	2		
• No eye opening	1		
Best verbal response			
• Oriented	5		
• Confused	4		4
• Inappropriate words	3		
• Incomprehensible sounds	2		
• No verbal response	1		
Best motor response			
• Obeys commands	6		6
• Localizes response to pain	5		
• Flexion withdrawal response to pain	4		
• Flexion abnormal response to pain	3		
• Extension response to pain	2		
• No motor response	1		
Total Glasgow Score			
• 13–15			14
• 9–12			
• 3–8			
• Other coma without documented GCS score or partial CGS score			

CHAPTER 4

Physician impression

1. AMS with confusion
2. Dehydration
3. Hyponatremia
4. Hyperkalemia
5. Acute kidney injury (AKI)
6. DM with hyperglycemia

QUERY: ALTERED MENTAL STATUS

Clinical indicators

1. "... significantly confused at the present time. She is oriented to self only; baseline mental status is unknown," per H&P, Dr. XXX 4/16/18

2. "... admitted with altered mental status most likely secondary to electrolyte imbalance and dehydration," per H&P, Dr. XXX 4/16/18

3. Neuro checks q two hours per MD orders 4/16/18

4. "No evidence of acute intracranial abnormalities. Diffuse microvascular chronic changes noted," per CT brain report 4/16/18

5. "Mentation: Confused, cooperative, GCS score 14," per physical exam, Dr. XXX 4/16/18

6. "... significantly confused at the present time. She is oriented to self only; baseline mental status is unknown," per H&P, Dr. XXX 4/16/18

7. "... admitted with altered mental status most likely secondary to electrolyte imbalance and dehydration," per H&P, Dr. XXX 4/16/18

8. Neuro checks q two hours per MD orders 4/16/18

9. "No evidence of acute intracranial abnormalities. Diffuse microvascular chronic changes noted," per CT brain report 4/16/18

10. "Mentation: Confused, cooperative, GCS score 14," per physical exam, Dr. XXX 4/16/18

CHAPTER 4

Request for clarification

Dr. XXX,

Please further specify the type and etiology of the altered mental status if known.

Thank you,
CDI Specialist, contact information

Options for response

- Dementia (please specify as pre-senile, senile, Alzheimer's, or other type)
- Electrolyte/metabolic imbalance (please specify)
- Encephalopathy
    - Diabetic
    - Metabolic
    - Other cause _____
    - Unable to determine or unknown
- Other condition (please specify) _____
- Unable to determine or unknown

CASE STUDIES: EXERCISES IN THE PRACTICAL APPLICATION OF THE CDI REVIEW PROCESS

Case study discussion: Altered mental status

AMS is a very common diagnosis that is more accurately described as a symptom of an underlying cause. The etiology of an alteration in mental status can be varied, and the CDI review should include an assessment of the testing and clinical findings from that testing. A leading expert in the field of clinical documentation is James S. Kennedy, MD, CCS, CDIP, CCDS, director at FTI Healthcare in Brentwood, Tennessee. Dr. Kennedy wrote in a 2009 white paper from the Association of Clinical Documentation Improvement Specialists (ACDIS) that, "in essence, altered mental status is to neurology what non-cardiac chest pain is to cardiology—a lower-weighted diagnosis whose severity improves with definition and documentation of the chronicity and nature of the symptom and the underlying cause."

An AMS can often be more clearly documented as delirium, dementia (stating the specific type of dementia as well), coma, or in terms of the Glasgow Coma Scale score. When educating your physicians, it is prudent to teach that terms such as confusion, disorientation, drowsy, or somnolence are simply symptom codes with little to no weight in determining acuity. It's important to note that AMS can result from organic brain disease or can be induced by external causes such as medications, poisons, or electrolyte disturbances.

Conversely, encephalopathy is coded as a diagnosis associated with a high severity and is the result of global brain dysfunction. According to Kennedy in the ACDIS white paper, "the best and most defendable definition of encephalopathy is published by the National Institutes of Health's National Institute of Neurological Disorders and Strokes." (The definition can be found at *www.ninds.nih.gov/disorders/encephalopathy/encephalopathy.htm*.)

"This publication defines encephalopathy as follows: Encephalopathy is a term for any diffuse disease of the brain that alters brain function or structure," Kennedy continues. "Encephalopathy may be caused by infectious agent (bacteria, virus, or prion), metabolic or mitochondrial dysfunction, brain tumor or increased pressure in the skull, prolonged exposure to toxic elements (including solvents, drugs, radiation, paints, industrial chemicals, and certain metals), chronic progressive trauma, poor nutrition, or lack of oxygen or blood flow to the brain."

"The hallmark of encephalopathy is an altered mental state. Depending on the type and severity of encephalopathy, common neurological symptoms are progressive loss of memory and cognitive ability, subtle personality changes, inability to concentrate, lethargy, and progressive loss of consciousness," Kennedy writes. "Other neurological symptoms may include myoclonus (involuntary twitching of a muscle or group of muscles), nystagmus (rapid, involuntary eye movement), tremor, muscle atrophy and weakness, dementia, seizures, and loss of ability to swallow or speak. Blood tests, spinal fluid examination, imaging studies, electroencephalograms, and similar diagnostic studies may be used to differentiate the various causes of encephalopathy."

If the clinical indicators, treatment, and test results clearly support the possible diagnosis of encephalopathy, then a query for that specificity should be posed to the physician.

It is crucial that the CDI specialist know and employ the following *Official Guidelines for Coding and Reporting* when performing medical record reviews:

> *For the Body Mass Index (BMI), depth of non-pressure chronic ulcers, pressure ulcer stage, coma scale, and NIH stroke scale (NIHSS) codes, code assignment may be based on medical record documentation from clinicians who are not the patient's provider (i.e., physician or other qualified healthcare practitioner legally accountable for establishing the patient's diagnosis), since this information is typically documented by other clinicians involved in the care of the patient (e.g., a dietitian often documents the BMI, a nurse often documents the pressure ulcer stages, and an emergency medical technician often documents the coma scale). However, the associated diagnosis (such as overweight, obesity, acute stroke, or pressure ulcer) must be documented by the patient's provider. If there is conflicting medical record documentation, either from the same clinician or different clinicians, the patient's attending provider should be queried for clarification.*

In any case where there is evidence of an alteration in mentation, the CDI specialist should look for evidence of standard assessment methods such as the GCS assessment. The GCS is scored between 3 and 15, with 3 being the worst, and 15 the best. It is composed of three parameters:

1. Best eye response

2. Best verbal response

3. Best motor response

Additional evaluation of the GCS score should incorporate the three distinct elements of the scoring. "Note that the phrase 'GCS of 11' is essentially meaningless, and it is important to break the figure down into its components, such as E3V3M5 = GCS 11," writes G. Teasdale and B. Jennette in *LANCET*. "A Coma Score of 13 or higher correlates with a mild brain injury, 9 to 12 is a moderate injury and 8 or less a severe brain injury."

CASE STUDIES: EXERCISES IN THE PRACTICAL APPLICATION OF THE CDI REVIEW PROCESS

Case Study: Hematology

Anemia

Physician documentation

History of present illness: The patient is a 48-year-old morbidly obese Caucasian female with debility, hypertension (HTN), end-stage renal disease (ESRD) on hemodialysis, chronic anemia, and depression. She is seen in the ED today with complaints of bloody stools, maroon in color, and generalized weakness. Denies any hematemesis.

Past medical history: ESRD, morbid obesity, functional debility, HTN, anemia of chronic kidney disease (CKD), depression. She is on hemodialysis with a Monday/Wednesday/Friday (MWF) schedule. She has experienced upper gastrointestinal (GI) bleed in the past due to a duodenal ulcer, treated with blood transfusions and clipping of the ulcer.

Home medications: Epogen, acetylsalicylic acid (ASA), Renagel, Lisinopril, Effexor

Physical exam:

- Vital signs: Afebrile, vital signs unremarkable
- Lungs: O_2 saturation is 100% on RA
- General: Abdomen, soft, obese, no tenderness noted
- BMI of 42
- Laboratory data from today revealed anemia of normocytic indexes

Treatment: GI consult for evaluation of source of rectal bleeding. Transfuse for hemoglobin (Hgb) < 7.0. Maintain hemodialysis on MWF schedule.

Clinical findings

Colonoscopy with upper endoscopy (EGD): Colonoscopy negative for evidence of lower GI bleed. EGD revealed a healing duodenal ulcer with no stigmata of active bleeding. The area around the duodenal ulcer was sensitive to the exam, however, and bled upon contact. The area was treated with a coagulator beam and bleeding ceased. Will transfuse packed red blood cells (PRBC) to attain Hgb of ≥ 7.0.

LABORATORY RESULTS

	Day 3	Day 2	Day 1
Hgb (g/dl)	8.3 (L)	8.9 (L)	6.2 (L)
Hct (%)	25.8 (L)	26.8 (L)	18.8 (L)
Platelets	213	180	228
RBC	2.95	3.09	2.88
Vitamin B12			358
BUN	53 (H)	46 (H)	48 (H)
Creatinine	4.0 (H)	3.8 (H)	3.9 (H)
GFR	<15 (L)	<15 (L)	<15 (L)
PT/INR			11.4/1.0

Impression

1. Recurrent gastrointestinal bleed due to duodenal ulcer; recent clipping of the duodenal ulcer

2. Anemia, transfused two units PRBC

3. ESRD, on hemodialysis

4. HTN

5. Morbid obesity

NOTES

QUERY: ANEMIA

Clinical indicators

1. "... Anemia of CKD ..." per H&P, Dr. Attending

2. "EGD revealed a healing duodenal ulcer with no stigmata of active bleeding. The area around the duodenal ulcer was sensitive to the exam, however, and bled upon contact," per EGD report, Dr. Gastroenterologist 4/20/18

3. "The area was treated with a coagulator beam and bleeding ceased," per EGD report, Dr. Gastroenterologist 4/20/18

4. "Anemia, transfused 2 units PRBC," per progress note, Dr. Gastroenterologist 4/20/18

5. Laboratory results:

	Day 3	Day 2	Day 1
Hgb (g/dl)	8.3 (L)	8.9 (L)	6.2 (L)
Hct (%)	25.8 (L)	26.8 (L)	18.8 (L)

Request for clarification

Dr. Attending,

Please specify the acuity and etiology of the anemia if known.

Thank you,

CDI Specialist, contact information

CHAPTER 4

Options for response

- Acuity:
  - Acute only
  - Chronic only
  - Acute on chronic combined
  - Other_____
  - Unable to determine_____

- Etiology:
  - Blood loss
  - End-stage renal disease
  - Combined etiology (specify the contributing conditions) _____
  - Other _____
  - Unable to determine _____

CASE STUDIES: EXERCISES IN THE PRACTICAL APPLICATION OF THE CDI REVIEW PROCESS

Case study discussion: Anemia

It's often a challenge for CDI specialists to obtain precise documentation of anemia in the medical record. A hospitalist once asked me why I sent him a query for anemia, as he said to me, "What difference does it make? I am going to treat it the same." That definitely got my documentation antennae up and I enthusiastically showed him all the various codes for anemia, the acuity, the etiology and, yes, even some different approaches to treatment, as not every anemia is treated with blood product transfusions.

So, why is it so difficult to get physicians to document anemia? While I'm not sure I have all the answers, I believe I can address at least some of the hesitancy. In my experience, surgeons are often reticent to document acute blood loss anemia from an overabundance of caution that this might reflect as a surgical complication. When you have the opportunity to discuss it with them, even if for only a few brief seconds, explain that a complication code is different from the acute blood loss anemia code. It can go a long way with your surgeons. Better yet, actually show them the complication code versus the acute blood loss anemia code. Factual presentation of data is often the best approach.

Another scenario where documentation of the "acute blood loss" component of the anemia diagnosis seems particularly difficult to pull from the documentation is in the situation where there is a gastrointestinal bleed, whether it be upper, lower, or both, as illustrated in this case study. Sometimes the physician is hesitant to declare the acute part of the diagnosis unless the patient is actively bleeding at the time of the colonoscopy or esophagogastroduodenoscopy (EGD). That's when our education mode kicks in to high gear when explaining that the use of terms such as probable, likely, or suspected is entirely appropriate for an inpatient encounter. And remind them to wrap it up nicely in the discharge summary for risk reduction for denial of payment.

I like to use my 15-second "elevator speech" whenever I have the opportunity to educate the physicians regarding documentation principles. An elevator speech is a brief and usually pre-scripted message that can be delivered impromptu to a physician as you are in the elevator or walking the corridor together. Practice your elevator speech so when the opportunity presents itself you are ready to spring into action.

CHAPTER 4

One example might be:

> *Hi, Dr. XXX! I just learned some interesting information about surgical complications. Did you know that a surgical complication must be explicitly documented as such, using terms like 'unexpected' or 'accidental' when describing the event? Otherwise, if the event is inherent to the procedure, that's not a complication.*

Okay, I just timed myself and I have to admit it took me 16.42 seconds to say all that! Still, you get the message. Just be prepared to drop your "pearls of wisdom" whenever you have the chance.

CASE STUDIES: EXERCISES IN THE PRACTICAL APPLICATION OF THE CDI REVIEW PROCESS

Case Study: Cardiovascular

Heart failure

Physician documentation

History of present illness: 72-year-old male presented to the ED with complaints of shortness of breath (SOB), leg swelling, and "heart racing in his chest" since early this morning. Denies chest pain or recent illness.

Past medical history: Includes a history of tobacco use, chronic obstructive pulmonary disease (COPD) with moderate pulmonary hypertension (PHTN), hyperlipidemia, congestive heart failure (CHF), atrial fibrillation, and noncompliance with prescription medications. Admits to continued tobacco smoking, and he has not refilled his medications for the past month due to financial hardship, with the exception of his Warfarin.

Home medications: Furosemide, Metoprolol, Amiodarone, Atorvastatin, Warfarin

Physical exam:

- Vital signs: BP in the ED was initially 162/88, HR 138, RR 30, afebrile
- 12-lead electrocardiogram (EKG) showed atrial fibrillation with rapid ventricular response ranging from 138–150
- O_2 saturation was 90% on RA and the patient was placed on 4 liters nasal cannula and O_2 saturation improved to 96%
- Lung: Anterior and posterior fields with rales in bilateral lower lobes

Treatment: 40 mg Furosemide IVP q 12 hours, stat portable chest X-ray (CXR), labs, and admit to telemetry unit. A Cardizem drip was begun and the BP was lowered to 142/82, HR decreased to 102 and RR decreased to 24. The EKG monitor showed atrial fibrillation with rate of 90–102.

Clinical findings

Radiology: Portable CXR report. There is cardiomegaly with slight prominence of the pulmonary vascular markings. These findings may represent CHF. Clinical correlation and imaging follow-up is advised.

Echocardiogram: A transthoracic bedside study was performed, with findings of decreased right ventricular function and ejection fraction (EF) of 30%.

Laboratory results: Include blood natriuretic peptide (BNP) 465, unremarkable complete blood count (CBC), negative metabolic panel, lactic acid 1.0, PT/INR 11.7/1.2, negative drug screen, and negative urinalysis.

Impression

1. Atrial fibrillation with rapid ventricular response
2. CHF
3. COPD, active tobacco smoker
4. Moderate pulmonary HTN
5. Noncompliant with medications

QUERY: HEART FAILURE

Clinical indicators

1. "c/o SOB, leg swelling," per H&P, Dr. Attending 3/01/18

2. History of "CHF," per H&P, Dr. Attending 3/01/18

3. "Lung fields with rales bilateral lower lobes," per H&P Dr. Attending 3/01/18

4. Furosemide 40 mg IVP in ER and then q 12 hours per MD orders and medication administration record

5. BNP 465 per labs 3/02/18

6. "...findings of decreased right ventricular function and ejection fraction of 30%," per Echo report 3/2/18

Request for clarification

Dr. Attending,

Please clarify the type, acuity, and etiology of the patient's CHF.

Thank you,
CDI Specialist, contact information

Options for response

- CHF type:
    - Systolic/heart failure with reduced ejection fraction (HFrEF)
    - Diastolic/heart failure with preserved ejection fraction (HFpEF)
    - Combined
    - Unable to determine
    - Other _____

- CHF acuity:
    - Acute
    - Chronic
    - Acute on chronic
    - Unable to determine
    - Other _____

- CHF etiology:
    - Hypertension
    - Other _____
    - Unable to determine

CASE STUDIES: EXERCISES IN THE PRACTICAL APPLICATION OF THE CDI REVIEW PROCESS

Case study discussion: Heart failure

The necessity for submitting a query to the provider for the specificity of heart failure seems to remain one of the leading reasons to query year after year, despite the efforts of CDI specialists to provide robust education around this diagnosis. The April 19, 2018, edition of *CDI Strategies* (the weekly electronic newsletter from ACDIS) revealed that CHF specificity and type topped the list of all queried diagnoses at a whopping 90.59% rate. Clearly, we still have a long way to go with educating our providers to document the complete diagnosis of congestive heart failure.

Heart failure is defined by the American College of Cardiology as a complex clinical syndrome that results from any structural or functional impairment of ventricular filling or ejection of blood. Systolic heart failure can also be documented as HFrEF while diastolic heart failure can also be documented as HFpEF.

When heart failure is the principal diagnosis, it drives the DRG to MS-DRG 291 (with an MCC), 292 (with a CC), or 293 (without an MCC or CC). While the specificity and type of heart failure will not change the DRG based on that information alone, it is still important to document the greatest specificity possible to ensure the highest level of accuracy in the medical record. Heart failure ICD-10 codes range from I50.1–I50.9 and include specificity for acuity and type. The etiology of the heart failure may direct you to an ICD-10 code outside of these. When the etiology is known, it is important to capture that in the documentation and coding. It's also important to note that heart failure is a CMS-Hierarchical Condition Category (HCC) for risk adjustment and stratification.

Terms such as "diastolic dysfunction" or "restrictive ventricular disease" are not synonymous with heart failure. When such terminology in the record is used interchangeably to indicate heart failure, the CDI specialist should query for the condition. Several clinical indicators are appropriate to use for clarification of heart failure, such as:

- BNP

- Echocardiogram results, including the ejection fraction percentage or terminology describing the nature of the heart failure

- Radiology findings that describe patterns or evidence of pulmonary vascular congestion, fluid accumulation, or a transudative pleural effusion

- Treatment with diuretics or fluid removal through dialysis

- Physical exam findings of jugular vein distention (JVD), extremity edema, or SOB

- Medications such as ACE inhibitors, beta-blockers, angiotensin II blockers (ARB), diuretics, and vasodilators; new drugs are constantly developed to treat heart failure, which affects nearly six million adults in the United States alone

CASE STUDIES: EXERCISES IN THE PRACTICAL APPLICATION OF THE CDI REVIEW PROCESS

Case Study: Nephrology

Case study: Chronic kidney disease

Physician documentation

History of present illness: An 89-year-old Hispanic female was admitted after an office visit to her primary care physician when abnormal labs were found with creatinine level of 2.4. The patient complains of nonproductive cough that is new onset for about two weeks, lower leg swelling, a four-pound weight gain this past week, and mild SOB. Denies noncompliance with medications.

Past medical history: History of CKD with mild elevation of creatinine but no acute symptomology, and renal function has been closely monitored and stable until now. Additional history of HTN, hyperlipidemia, atrial fibrillation, and aortic valvular disease with transcatheter aortic valve replacement (TAVR) two months ago.

Home medications: Bumex, Norvasc, Simvastatin, Warfarin, potassium chloride

Physical exam:

- Heart: controlled rate and irregular rhythm
- Vascular: BLE 3+ edema
- Vital signs—128/60, 88, 20, afebrile, O_2 sat 97% on room air

Treatment: Admit to telemetry, IV Lasix BID and closely monitor renal function, cardiology and nephrology consults, echo, CT of abdomen without contrast to preserve renal function, and bilateral lower extremity Doppler ultrasound.

Clinical findings

Radiology: CXR report stated acute pulmonary edema with small pleural effusions.

LE Doppler ultrasound: Negative for occlusion, bilateral lower extremities.

Echocardiogram: TAVR in place and functioning normally. Left atrium severely enlarged. Left ventricle size, function, and structure appear within normal limits.

CT abdomen: Negative for acute findings.

LABORATORY RESULTS

	Day 5	Day 4	Day 3	Day 2	Day 1
Blood urea nitrogen (BUN)	49 (H)	52 (H)	50 (H)	53 (H)	56 (H)
Creatinine	2.4 (H)	2.6 (H)	2.4 (H)	2.4 (H)	2.4 (H)
Glomerular filtration rate (GFR)	25.8 (L)	23.5 (L)	25.6 (L)	25.7 (L)	24.8 (L)
BNP				422 (H)	945 (H)

Impression

1. Acute on chronic diastolic congestive heart failure
2. Acute kidney injury
3. CKD
4. HTN
5. Chronic atrial fibrillation with controlled rate
6. Status post (S/P) TAVR

NOTES

QUERY: CHRONIC KIDNEY DISEASE

Clinical indicators

1. "Chronic Kidney Disease" per nephrology consult note 2/25

2. "History of CKD with mild elevation of creatinine, but no acute symptomology and renal function has been closely monitored and stable until now," per H&P 2/25

3. "CT abdomen without contrast to preserve renal function," per MD orders 2/26

4. Laboratory findings:

	Day 5	Day 4	Day 3	Day 2	Day 1
BUN	49	52	50	53	56
Creatinine	2.4	2.6	2.4	2.4	2.4
GFR	25.8	25.0	25.6	25.7	24.8

Request for clarification:

Dr. Nephrologist,

Please further specify the stage of the CKD if known.

Thank you,
CDI Specialist, contact information

Options for response

- CKD Stage 1
- CKD Stage 2 (mild)
- CKD Stage 3 (moderate)
- CKD Stage 4 (severe)
- CKD Stage 5
- ESRD
- Other _____
- Unable to determine/unknown _____

CASE STUDIES: EXERCISES IN THE PRACTICAL APPLICATION OF THE CDI REVIEW PROCESS

Case study discussion: Chronic kidney disease

CKD is coded according to severity, and it's stratified into five progressive stages and a final sixth category of ESRD. Definitions for the different stages are described by the National Kidney Foundation as:

- **Stage 1:** GFR 90+, normal kidney function but urine findings or structural abnormalities or genetic traits point to kidney disease

- **Stage 2:** GFR 60–89, mildly reduced kidney function, and other findings (as for stage 1) point to kidney disease

- **Stage 3:** GFR 30–59, moderately reduced kidney function

- **Stage 4:** GFR 15–29, severely reduced kidney function

- **Stage 5:** ESRD with GFR < 15, very severe, or end-stage kidney failure not yet requiring dialysis

- **ESRD:** End-stage renal disease with GFR < 15, very severe, or end-stage kidney failure requiring chronic dialysis

Renal disease often accompanies conditions such as DM and HTN. ICD-10-CM coding guidelines instruct coding professionals to assume the causal relationship between CKD and HTN (unless the provider specifically states that the two conditions are not related), as well as in the case of CKD and diabetes mellitus (unless the provider specifically states that the two conditions are not related).

According to an article in the *American Journal of Medicine,* "the co-morbid conditions of DM and HTN present the dominant risk factors for CKD." The relevance of capturing these conditions to the greatest degree of specificity possible cannot be overemphasized, and the astute CDI specialist will maintain awareness that CKD at any stage is a CMS-HCC for risk adjustment and stratification.

Terminolgy such as "avoid nephrotoxic drugs," "adminstration of fluids," or "Mucomyst prior to procedures involving the administration of dye" are clues to the CDI specialist to look closer for additional indicators that may signal CKD.

CHAPTER 4

Case Study: Procedures

Case study: Debridement

Physician documentation

History of present illness: The patient is a 71-year-old Asian female with a past medical history (PMH) of non-insulin-dependent DM (NIDDM) and HTN who presents with a two-day history of left groin pain with fevers and chills. The patient denies any lesion, cut, trauma, wounds, or insect bite to the groin area.

Previous medical history: Relatively healthy Asian female with a history of HTN on Lisinopril 5 mg daily and has DM treated with Metformin daily.

Home medications: Lisinopril, Metformin. The patient has been taking acetaminophen to relieve the groin and LLQ abdominal pain. Also, she states that she took some "leftover" antibiotics from a previous infection but is unable to recall the name of the antibiotic or what it was prescribed for.

Physical exam:

- Left groin area tender and hot to the touch with + fluctuance
- Vital signs: Temperature 102.6° F; 110/68; HR 92; RR 18; O_2 saturation 99% on 2 liters per nasal cannula
- Heart—Negative
- Lungs—Negative
- Neuro—Alert and oriented ×3
- Integumentary—Left groin and LLQ abdomen are tender, painful
- Posterior tibial and dorsalis pedis pulses 3 + bilaterally

Treatment: CT abdomen and pelvis, left lower extremity venous Doppler study, general surgery consult, broad-spectrum antibiotics.

CASE STUDIES: EXERCISES IN THE PRACTICAL APPLICATION OF THE CDI REVIEW PROCESS

Surgery consult:

- Preoperative: Suspected necrotizing fasciitis of left groin. Will take to OR for exploration, possible incision and drainage (I&D), and further treatment as indicated.

- Postoperative: Necrotizing fasciitis, debridement of all necrotic tissue. Wound vacuum applied. Continue with wound vacuum and broad-spectrum antibiotic coverage; wound cultures pending.

Operative/procedure note

Procedure: I&D and sharp debridement of left thigh.

The patient was brought to the operating room and placed on the table in the supine position and a timeout was performed. The left thigh and groin were prepped in the usual sterile manner. As I made the incision over the area of fluctuance, there was immediate malodorous drainage. The drainage was cultured. Extensive sharp debridement was performed and all necrotic tissue was removed. A wound vacuum was placed. The patient tolerated the procedure well, with vital signs stable throughout and estimated blood loss (EBL) was <10 ml.

Clinical findings

CT abdomen and pelvis with contrast: Findings of an area of soft tissue gas in the left upper thigh extending to the mons pubis area with no evidence of abscess. Clinical correlation is recommended for further assessment.

Lower extremity venous Doppler: Negative for deep vein thrombosis (DVT) or venous circulatory compromise.

Surgical pathology report: Left groin skin and subcutaneous tissue with significant acute and chronic inflammation and necrosis with abscess formation.

LABORATORY RESULTS

	Day 14	Day 12	Day 10	Day 8	Day 6	Day 4	Day 3	Day 2	Day 1
Lactic acid								1.6	1.8
WBC	4.1 (L)	4.4 (L)	3.9 (L)	4.8 (L)	4.8 (L)	5.0 (L)	13.0 (H)	13.9 (H)	13.2 (H)
Neutrophils	38.4 (L)	31.3 (L)	33.6 (L)	34.0 (L)	38.7 (L)	37.9 (L)	86.1 (H)	87.9 (H)	88.3 (H)
Platelets	144 (L)	150 (L)	142 (L)	155 (L)	150 (L)	138 (L)	88 (L)	77 (L)	79 (L)
Blood glucose	110 (H)	129 (H)	118 (H)	136 (H)	124 (H)	235 (H)	106 (H)	168 (H)	342 (H)
HIV screen									Negative
Hepatitis screen									Negative

Impression

1. Necrotizing fasciitis, left thigh
2. Fever
3. Leukocytosis
4. DM, type 2

Procedure

1. I&D and sharp debridement of left thigh with wound vacuum placement

NOTES

CASE STUDIES: EXERCISES IN THE PRACTICAL APPLICATION OF THE CDI REVIEW PROCESS

QUERY: DEBRIDEMENT

Clinical indicators

1. "Incision and drainage and sharp debridement of left thigh with wound vacuum placement," per operative procedure note, Dr. General Surgeon on 3/15/18

2. "Extensive sharp debridement was performed and all necrotic tissue was removed," per Operative Procedure note, Dr. XXX on 3/15/18

Request for clarification

Dr. General Surgeon,

Please specify the type of debridement performed, the instrumentation used and the deepest level of tissue removed.

Thank you,
CDI Specialist, contact information

Options for response

Procedure:

- Excisional (surgical removal/cutting away of devitalized tissue, necrosis, or slough).
    - Type of instrument used
    - Deepest level of tissue removed
        - Skin
        - Subcutaneous
        - Muscle

- Fascia

- Bone

- Other _____

• Nonexcisional debridement (nonsurgical snipping, brushing, irrigation, scrubbing or washing of devitalized tissue, necrosis, or slough)

- Type of instrument used

- Deepest level of tissue removed

- Skin

- Subcutaneous

- Muscle

- Fascia

- Bone

- Other _____

Case study discussion: Debridement

CDI specialists often find that documentation concerning a debridement can be confusing and lacking in the specificity necessary to accurately code the procedure. There is a lot of confusion among providers as well, and oftentimes the provider believes the specificity provided in the procedure note is more than adequate. The coding of debridement, however, is more complex and requires a standard of specificity that is very well defined.

Debridement is defined as "the removal of foreign material or devitalized tissue from or adjacent to a traumatic or infected lesion until surrounding healthy tissue is exposed." It can be performed on skin, subcutaneous tissue, fascia, muscle, or bone.

A second definition of debridement goes more in depth:

> *Debridement is the surgical removal of contaminated or devitalized subcutaneous/fascia/muscle/ bone tissue or foreign matter that is damaged, necrotic, dead, infected, abscessed, or ischemic, caused by injury, infection, wounds (excluding burn wounds), or chronic ulcers. Using a scalpel or dermatome, the physician excises the affected subcutaneous tissue until viable, bleeding tissue is encountered.*

When the CDI specialist reviews a record that includes a debridement, it is important to look for clues in the terminology that can assist in determining the specifics of the procedure. Terms such as "sharp debridement" do not suffice or equate to the term excisional. Words such as sharp, bone, wound, muscle, ulcer, necrosis, slough, and similar terminology are clues for the CDI specialist to review the record in greater detail to determine the true condition and procedure being addressed.

The term excisional must meet the root operation term in ICD-10-Procedural coding system (ICD-10-PCS) of "excision," which is defined as the "cutting out or off, without replacement, a portion of a body part." A debridement may be performed on any body part and may occur in the operating room suite, the bedside, or in a whirlpool. Aside from a physician, there are other healthcare professionals who are qualified to perform a debridement, including wound care nurses, physical therapists, and nurse practitioners.

CHAPTER 4

The coding definition of a "nonexcisional debridement includes brushing, irrigating or washing of devitalized tissue, necrosis or slough." A nonexcisional debridement is not considered a valid operating room procedure and will not move the MS-DRG to a surgical DRG.

When reviewing a record with a debridement, the CDI specialist should carefully review the operative or procedure note to determine whether the documentation clearly describes the type of debridement (excisional versus nonexcisional), the depth of the debridement (up to and including which type of tissue), and the instrumentation used to perform the procedure. Note that the often abbreviated "I & D" procedure may need additional clarification by means of a query to the performing provider. The "D" may represent the term drainage or it may represent the term debridement. Careful review of the body of the procedure note may be necessary to determine the true procedure performed, with a query presented in cases where it is unclear.

CASE STUDIES: EXERCISES IN THE PRACTICAL APPLICATION OF THE CDI REVIEW PROCESS

Case Study: Nutrition

Case study: Malnutrition

Physician documentation

History of present illness: An 80-year-old Caucasian female is admitted to the hospital after her husband and daughter brought her to the ED, stating that she is refusing to eat and is becoming weaker and less responsive. The patient appears cachectic and dehydrated with dry mucous membranes, sunken orbital areas, and thready, but weak and faintly palpable pedal pulses. Family states she has refused all food and fluids for two days now.

Past medical history: History of atrial fibrillation for 25 years after she contacted a viral infection. No history of coronary artery disease (CAD), angina, or myocardial infarction. No history of heart failure. History of DM type 2, treated with oral medications and diet. Never used insulin. Previous tobacco smoker with 40-pack-a-year history. Quit smoking more than 20 years ago. History of Parkinson's disease with progressive debility over the past 10 years. Patient is now bed-bound and requires all activities of daily life (ADL) performed for her. Her husband is the primary caregiver with occasional assistance from skilled nursing assistants. Her husband was recently diagnosed with end-stage pancreatic cancer with metastases to liver and lungs. Her daughter is a nurse and lives out of state; her son lives locally.

Home medications: Warfarin, Metformin, Levodopa

Physical exam:

- Heart: Irregular rhythm with rate 94.
- Lungs: Shallow breaths, decreased breath sounds anterior and posterior, bilaterally.
- Vital signs: BP 114/68, HR 94, RR 16, temperature 98.0°F, height 68", weight 102 pounds, GCS 13.
- Integumentary: Skin cool, dry, no skin breakdown noted but bruising on bony prominences as is typical of anticoagulant therapy.
- Neurological: Somnolent, responsive to verbal stimuli. Oriented to name, disoriented to place and time. Knows husband and children. Cooperative with requests. Parkinson tremors visible and head-bobbing observed. Hand grip weak to almost nonexistent.

Treatment: Admit to general medical floor. Dietary consult. Will ask her neurologist and cardiologist to consult. IV fluids, labs, CXR, echo pending update from her cardiologist. Will pursue palliative care consult after discussion with the family.

Clinical findings

Radiology: Portable CXR: Difficult study as patient is unable to sit upright to assess lung expansion. No acute evidence of infiltrate or fluid consolidation. Bilateral bases with minimal expansion and suspected significant atelectasis. No evidence of COPD despite smoking history.

Dietary consult notes: Patient with history of Parkinson's disease with progressive debility. Husband is primary caretaker and recently diagnosed with terminal cancer. Patient stated to me that she does not want to live without her husband and she will not eat or drink anymore. Patient stated she does not want a feeding tube and does not want to prolong her life. Recommend ice chips, popsicles, and oral hygiene for comfort. Nutritional assessment: severe protein calorie deficit due to chronic debilitating disease with progressive decrease in function and loss of will to live. BMI is 15.51 with severe loss of muscle mass, very weak handgrip, and temporal wasting evident. Will discuss findings and patient's statements to me with her attending physician.

LABORATORY RESULTS

	Day 3	Day 2	Day 1
BUN	35 (H)	36 (H)	38.2 (H)
Creatinine	2.9 (H)	3.1 (H)	3.2 (H)
GFR	30.1 (L)	32.2 (L)	36.4 (L)
UA specific gravity			1.065 (H)
UA color			Dark amber (Abnormal)
NA+	132 (L)	132 (L)	130 (L)
K+	4.0	4.8	5.2
CL−	108 (H)	109 (H)	110 (H)
CO_2	19 (L)	18 (L)	18 (L)
Glucose	99	109	104
Total protein	5.0 (L)	5.4 (L)	5.5 (L)
WBC	8.1 (L)	8.0 (L)	8.2 (L)
Hgb	15.0 (H)	15.3 (H)	16.0 (H)
Hct	44.1 (H)	44.9 (H)	45.4 (H)
Platelets	316	312	320

CHAPTER 4

GLASGOW COMA SCALE

	GCS score	Day 1 score
Eye opening		
• Spontaneous	4	
• Response to verbal command	3	3
• Response to pain	2	
• No eye opening	1	
Best verbal response		
• Oriented	5	
• Confused	4	4
• Inappropriate words	3	
• Incomprehensible sounds	2	
• No verbal response	1	
Best motor response		
• Obeys commands	6	6
• Localizes response to pain	5	
• Flexion withdrawal response to pain	4	
• Flexion abnormal response to pain	3	
• Extension response to pain	2	
• No motor response	1	
Total Glasgow Score		
• 13–15		13
• 9–12		
• 3–8		
• Other coma without documented GCS score or partial CGS score		

CASE STUDIES: EXERCISES IN THE PRACTICAL APPLICATION OF THE CDI REVIEW PROCESS

Impression:

1. Dehydration
2. Parkinson's disease
3. AMS
4. Debility
5. DM 2
6. Atrial fibrillation with controlled ventricular response
7. Failure to thrive

NOTES

CHAPTER 4

QUERY: MALNUTRITION

Clinical indicators:

1. "... she is refusing to eat and is becoming weaker and less responsive," per H&P, Dr. Attending

2. "Patient appears cachectic and dehydrated..." per H&P, Dr. Attending

3. "Nutritional assessment: severe protein calorie deficit due to chronic debilitating disease with progressive decrease in function and loss of will to live," per registered dietitian consult notes on 6/10/18

4. "BMI is 15.51 with severe loss of muscle mass, very weak handgrip, and temporal wasting evident," per registered dietitian consult notes on 6/10/18

5. "Failure to thrive," per H&P, Dr. Attending

Request for clarification:

Dr. Attending,

Can the nutritional status be further specified?

Thank you,
CDI Specialist, contact information

CASE STUDIES: EXERCISES IN THE PRACTICAL APPLICATION OF THE CDI REVIEW PROCESS

Options for response:

- Failure to thrive (adult)
- Malnutrition
    - Mild/first degree
    - Moderate/second degree
    - Severe/third degree
- No malnutrition
- Other _____
- Unable to determine

CHAPTER 4

Case study discussion: Malnutrition

In April 2012, the Academy of Nutrition and Dietetics and the American Society for Parenteral and Enteral Nutrition (ASPEN) jointly published a consensus statement commonly referred to as the ASPEN paper. The consensus statement is considered by many to be the leading reference in assessing adult malnutrition, but it is not universally accepted as such, so debate continues across the healthcare continuum.

In the paper, ASPEN asserts that:

> *Adult malnutrition is a common but frequently unrecognized problem whose incidence and prevalence are difficult to determine. In 1996, The Joint Commission mandated that nutrition screening be accomplished within 24 hours of admission. This resulted in the identification of multiple criteria and the development of a number of different approaches to the identification of malnutrition in hospitalized patients that were not always evidence based. Thus, there is currently no single, universally accepted approach to the diagnosis and documentation of adult malnutrition.*

The following can serve as clinical indicators for a malnutrition query or may provide the impetus to looker deeper in the record for more information:

- Weight loss.
- Diminished muscle mass, subcutaneous fat loss.
- Impaired wound healing.
- Temporal wasting.
- BMI < 19; however, it is important to note that malnutrition may occur at any BMI, not just below 19. A patient who is obese can still suffer from malnutrition when protein calorie intake is insufficient to meet the demands of the body.
- Feeding tube, supplemental feedings, parenteral nutrition.
- Dry, thin skin with poor turgor.
- Dry brittle nails and hair.
- Loss of skin pigmentation.
- Anemia.

CASE STUDIES: EXERCISES IN THE PRACTICAL APPLICATION OF THE CDI REVIEW PROCESS

- Chronic diseases.

- Generalized fluid accumulation or edema that could mask weight loss.

- Dietary consult and all associated notes, insufficient protein calorie intake.

- Depression, apathy, weakness, cachexia, diminished hand grip strength.

- Serum albumin and pre-albumin are not diagnostic criteria for malnutrition. (These are proteins that will reflect a decrease when faced with trauma, burns, or SIRS.)

A word of caution about the malnutrition code E40, Kwashiorkor: This condition is extremely rare in a developed country such as the United States and should be used very judiciously, if at all. A recent article in *CDI Strategies* (ACDIS' weekly electronic newsletter) notes that, "The diagnosis of malnutrition has long been in the sights of the Office of Inspector General (OIG) for audits and denials. In fact, just as recently as December 2017, the OIG found that of 2,145 inpatient claims from 2006–2014 at 25 providers, all but one incorrectly included the diagnosis code for kwashiorkor. This resulted in overpayments in excess of $6 million."

CHAPTER 4

Case Study: Multiple Conditions

Case study

Physician documentation

History of present illness: The patient is a 90-year-old African-American female who had apparently been down for an unknown period of time. The patient's daughter found her on the kitchen floor and unresponsive and she called 911. When the paramedics arrived the patient was unresponsive with a blood glucose level in the low 30s, severe bradycardia with a HR of 40, and agonal respirations. The patient was given glucose and was intubated, had transcutaneous pacing, and was brought into our facility. C-spine precautions taken due to possible unwitnessed fall.

Past medical history: History obtained from daughter: HTN, diabetes mellitus, CHF, CAD, transient ischemic attack (TIA), pneumonia.

Home medications: Glipizide, Metoprolol, Lasix

Physical exam:

- Heart: Regular rhythm at rate of 56. Transcutaneous pacemaker pads in place for continued sinus bradycardia. No AV block noted. 12-lead EKG negative for acute ST segment elevated myocardial infarction (STEMI).

- Lungs: Intubated on mechanical ventilation with decreased breath sounds bilateral bases. ETT position confirmed via CXR. ? aspiration given the altered mental status upon admission.

- Integumentary: No obvious cuts, abrasions, lacerations. Skin hot and dry. Appears dehydrated.

- Renal: Foley catheter placed with 60 ml concentrated urine returned.

- Vital signs: Temperature 101.4°F rectal; BP 94/66 on vasopressor support; Goal MAP ≥60; HR 56-68; RR 16, ventilator dependent; O_2 saturation 99% on 80% FiO_2; Ht. 62 inches; wt. 112 lbs.; BMI 20.48; GCS score 5 in ED.

CASE STUDIES: EXERCISES IN THE PRACTICAL APPLICATION OF THE CDI REVIEW PROCESS

Treatment: The patient was found to be hypotensive in the ED, was started on vasopressors, and has been admitted to the intensive care unit (ICU). Sepsis protocol initiated. The patient was also found to have renal insufficiency and nephrology has been consulted. Pulmonary consulted for ventilator management and possible PNA. Neurology has been consulted for AMS and evaluation of possible TIA/cerebrovascular accident (CVA). Ultrasound of the kidneys, echocardiogram. IV fluids for rhabdomyolysis. Broad-spectrum antibiotics. Blood, sputum, and urine cultures. Continue mechanical ventilation; decrease FiO_2 to 80%, rate of 16, tidal volume 500, PEEP 5. SCDs and GI prophylaxis. CT to assess for fractures, brain injury.

Clinical findings

Radiology: CT of brain negative for bleed. CT of body negative for acute fractures.

CXR: Bilateral atelectasis lower lobes. Consolidation noted right lung, suspicious for pneumonia. Correlate with clinical findings.

Echocardiogram: Global hypokinesis, left ventricular hypertrophy, EF 35%.

Renal ultrasound: Evidence of hydronephrosis, kidneys bilaterally are small in size.

CHAPTER 4

LABORATORY RESULTS

	Day 3	Day 2	Day 1
ABG on admission			Ph 7.20, pCO$_2$ 32, pO$_2$ 143, HCO$_3$ 7.3, Base Excess −22 (on 100% FiO$_2$ per AMBU in ED)
WBC	10.4 (H)	13.8 (H)	14.1 (H)
Hgb	9.9 (L)	11.1 (L)	12.8
Hct	28.6 (L)	33.5	39.8
Platelets	250	280	309
Neutrophils	98 (H)	88 (H)	83 (H)
Urinalysis			Positive for UTI, muddy casts, high specific gravity
Na+	136	134 (L)	129 (L)
K+	4.8	5.2 (H)	6.4 (H)
CL−	101	103	95 (L)
CO$_2$	18	18	8 (L)
BUN	49 (H)	57 (H)	59 (H)
Creatinine	6.56 (H)	8.9 (H)	9.58 (H)
GFR	45.6 (L)	33.6 (L)	31.2 (L)
CK	1,500	2,407	4,108
Ammonia		30	32
Blood glucose	140 (H)	118	78 after treatment by EMS prior to arrival in ER (L)
Drug screen			Negative
Lactic acid	2.6 (H)	4.2 (H)	4.8 (H)
Blood CX	Pending @ 48 hrs.	Pending	Pending
Urine CX	+ E.coli	Pending	Pending
Sputum CX	+ Pseudomonas	Pending	Pending

CASE STUDIES: EXERCISES IN THE PRACTICAL APPLICATION OF THE CDI REVIEW PROCESS

GLASGOW COMA SCALE

	GCS score	Day 2 score	Day 1 score
Eye opening			
• Spontaneous	4		
• Response to verbal command	3		
• Response to pain	2		
• No eye opening	1	1	1
Best verbal response			
• Oriented	5		
• Confused	4		
• Inappropriate words	3		
• Incomprehensible sounds	2		
• No verbal response	1	1	1
Best motor response			
• Obeys commands	6		
• Localizes response to pain	5		
• Flexion withdrawal response to pain	4		
• Flexion abnormal response to pain	3	3	3
• Extension response to pain	2		
• No motor response	1		
Total Glasgow Score			
• 13–15			
• 9–12			
• 3–8		5	5
• Other coma without documented GCS score or partial CGS score			

CHAPTER 4

Impression

1. Acute respiratory distress
2. Metabolic acidosis
3. Acute renal insufficiency
4. Rhabdomyolysis
5. Acute metabolic and septic encephalopathy
6. Shock
7. History of CHF and prior history of stenting, CAD
8. Leukocytosis
9. Hyperkalemia and hyponatremia

NOTES

QUERY: PNEUMONIA SPECIFICITY

Clinical indicators

1. "Pulmonary consulted for ventilator management and possible PNA," per H&P, Dr. XXX 6/17/18

2. "Consolidation noted right lung, suspicious for pneumonia. Correlate with clinical findings," per CXR report 6/17/18

3. "? aspiration given the AMS upon admission," per progress note, Dr. XXX 6/17/18

4. "Broad-spectrum antibiotics," per Dr. XXX orders and progress note 6/17/18

5. Sputum culture + for pseudomonas on day 3 of hospitalization

Request for clarification

Dr. XXX,

Please clarify if this patient is being treated for suspected or confirmed pneumonia. If yes, please further specify the type of pneumonia if known.

Thank you,
CDI Specialist, contact information

Options for response

- No pneumonia

- Pneumonia

    – Gram positive (please specify the organism, if known)

    – Gram negative (please specify the organism, if known)

    – Aspiration pneumonia (please document the specific aspirate, if known)

    – Bacterial pneumonia (please specify the organism, if known)

- Other _____

- Unable to determine/unknown

CASE STUDIES: EXERCISES IN THE PRACTICAL APPLICATION OF THE CDI REVIEW PROCESS

QUERY: RESPIRATORY FAILURE

Clinical indicators

1. "Acute respiratory distress," per H&P impression, Dr. XXX 5/1/18

2. "Lungs: intubated on mechanical ventilation with decreased breath sounds bilateral bases. ETT position confirmed via CXR," per H&P physical exam, Dr. XXX 5/1/18

3. Arterial blood gas (ABG) on admission to ED 5/1/18 at 1640, 100% FiO_2 per Ambu assist:

pH	7.20
pCO_2	32
pO_2	143
HCO_3-	7.8
Base excess	−22

Request for clarification

Dr. XXX,

Please further document the specificity and the acuity of the patient's respiratory condition being treated.

Thank you,
CDI specialist, contact information

Options for response

- Diagnosis:
  - Dyspnea
  - Respiratory insufficiency
  - Respiratory failure
  - Other (please specify) _____
  - Unable to determine/unknown

- Acuity:
  - Acute
  - Chronic
  - Combined acute on chronic
  - Other (please specify) _____
  - Unable to determine/unknown

- Associated conditions:
  - With hypercapnia
  - With hypoxia
  - With combined hypercapnia and hypoxia
  - Other (please specify) _____
  - Unable to determine/unknown

QUERY: ACUTE KIDNEY INJURY

Clinical indicators

1. "Acute renal insufficiency," per impression, H&P, Dr. XXX 6/17/18

2. "Appears dehydrated," per H&P, Dr. XXX 6/17/18

3. "IV fluids for rhabdomyolysis," per H&P, Dr. XXX 6/17/18

4. "Evidence of hydronephrosis, kidneys bilaterally are small in size," per renal US 6/18/18

5. Laboratory findings:

	Day 3	Day 2	Day 1
BUN	49 (H)	57 (H)	59 (H)
Creatinine	6.56 (H)	8.9 (H)	9.58 (H)
GFR	45.6 (L)	33.6 (L)	31.2 (L)

Request for clarification

Dr. XXX,

Please further specify the patient's acute renal insufficiency and the etiology if known.

Thank you,
CDI Specialist, contact information

CHAPTER 4

Options for response

- Acute kidney condition:

    – Acute renal insufficiency/disorder of kidney and ureter, unspecified

    – Acute kidney failure, unspecified

    – Acute kidney failure with tubular necrosis

    – Other _____

    – Unable to determine/unknown

- Underlying cause:

    – Dehydration

    – Rhabdomyolysis

    – Shock (please specify the type of shock)

    – Other _____

    – Unable to determine/unknown

CASE STUDIES: EXERCISES IN THE PRACTICAL APPLICATION OF THE CDI REVIEW PROCESS

QUERY: INFECTION SPECIFICITY

Clinical indicators

1. "Sepsis protocol initiated," per Dr. XXX orders and H&P 6/18/18

2. "Started on vasopressors and has been admitted to intensive care unit," per Dr. XXX H&P 6/18/18

3. "Acute metabolic and septic encephalopathy," per H&P impression, Dr. XXX 6/18/18

4. "Shock," per H&P impression, Dr. XXX 6/18/18

5. Laboratory results:

	Day 3	Day 2	Day 1
WBC	10.4	13.8	14.1
Neutrophils	98	88	83
Urinalysis			Positive for UTI, muddy casts, high specific gravity
Lactic acid	2.6	4.2	4.8
Blood CX	Pending @ 48 hrs.	Pending	Pending
Urine CX	+ E.coli	Pending	Pending
Sputum CX	+ Pseudomonas	Pending	Pending

CHAPTER 4

Request for clarification

Dr. XXX,

Is there a diagnosis associated with the above-listed clinical indicators? If yes, please further specify the condition to the greatest degree possible.

Thank you,
CDI Specialist, contact information

Options for response

- Bacteremia
- Sepsis (specify degree of severity and the etiology if known)
    - Severe sepsis
    - Severe sepsis due to _____
    - Severe sepsis with septic shock due to _____
- Localized infectious process only
- Urinary tract infection (specify organism if known)
- Pneumonia (specify organism if known)
- Other (please specify) _____
- Unable to determine

CASE STUDIES: EXERCISES IN THE PRACTICAL APPLICATION OF THE CDI REVIEW PROCESS

Case study discussion: Multiple diagnoses

The seasoned CDI specialist who encounters a case scenario like the one described here will be challenged to critically analyze several aspects of the case, multiple concurrent conditions, as well as an often rapidly evolving clinical picture. Some of the elements of the review are obvious and the CDI specialist can easily focus on those diagnoses that need further clarification. When faced with multiple body systems that are affected, however, a sound clinical foundation is essential to a thorough and complete review. A deep fundamental knowledge of pathophysiology and acute care medicine will serve the CDI specialist well in a complex review such as this.

As we know, not all is crystal clear and definitive in medicine. It can truly be like the proverbial case of which came first, the chicken or the egg? There are many situations in which physicians piece together the known facts of a patient's illness and then complement that knowledge with hypothetical models that may explain, totally or in part, the clinical picture and the response to treatment that is evidenced.

As the CDI specialist reviews the information presented in this case, there are key factors that should stand out to prompt the investigative process that is central to an expert CDI review. This scenario starts with a patient that was found down for an unknown period of time, from an unknown etiology, and with multiple critical and life-threatening conditions. As the CDI specialist examines the records, there are several questions that should surface.

Overview

A good place to begin is in determining if documentation or clinical evidence exists that points to the etiology of the episode. The patient has a history of DM with a blood glucose level at the scene in the low 30s. Was this a possible etiology or perhaps an adverse effect of diabetes medication? The patient was found down on the floor. Did the patient fall as a result of tripping or did another event precede the fall? Did the patient's low blood glucose level cause the patient to experience a syncopal episode and then fall, or did the fall trigger the blood glucose drop to dangerous levels after ingestion of the diabetes medication but before the patient had eaten? The CDI specialist should conduct the record review with these questions in mind, searching for clues to the answers that will determine whether the documentation aligns with the clinical picture.

The patient also has a history of TIAs. Is there evidence of a TIA or cerebrovascular accident? What are the results of the computed tomography (CT) scan? Was a magnetic resonance imaging (MRI) scan done, and if so what are the results? Since there appears to have been a traumatic fall, it is important to assess the brain for evidence of bleeding. Additionally, the patient has a history of HTN and there exists the possibility that this could have resulted from a hypertensive episode that in turn caused cerebral hemorrhage. A CT scan of the brain done upon arrival should reflect evidence of brain hemorrhage if present. However, it may take days for evidence of an ischemic or thrombotic CVA to appear on a MRI study.

Additionally, scanning the patient for fractures elsewhere in the body is indicated. It was noted in the documentation that C-spine precautions were observed to protect the patient from possible further injury. With the results of the CT and MRI imaging scans negative for acute CVA, negative for spinal injury, and negative for fractures, the CDI specialist can move on to other aspects of the case.

Pneumonia specificity

Next, the CDI specialist may turn attention to respiratory conditions; the agonal respirations and subsequent intubation that followed when paramedics arrived on the scene. Given the unresponsive state and unknown circumstances that led to the event, the CDI specialist should focus on the high risk for this patient to have experienced an aspiration event. The documentation in the record states "unknown aspiration given the altered mental status upon admission." The CXR report reflects "consolidation in the right lung, suspicious for pneumonia." When a review of the treatment for the "unknown aspiration" and the "possible pneumonia" reflected in the physician's treatment plan, the CDI specialist should look for evidence of the type of pneumonia.

Investigating the microbiology lab results (sputum culture) that could reflect the offending organism being treated is warranted. It is important to note at this point that there are some basic tenets that the CDI specialist should remain mindful of: While sputum culture results of a specific organism such as *Klebsiella pneumoniae, Pseudomonas,* or perhaps *Staphylococcus aureus* (all are Gram-negative organisms) are beneficial in determining appropriate antibiotic coverage targeted at the specific organism, the absence of such definitive results does not preclude a diagnosis of Gram-negative pneumonia. The microbiology lab results in this case grew *Pseudomonas*; therefore, documentation of the offending organism with the concurrent Gram-negative antibiotic coverage could result in a more precise diagnosis of pneumonia due to *Pseudomonas*.

Aspiration pneumonia is coded as pneumonitis and can be due to solids or liquids, inhalation of food and vomit, or inhalation of other solids and liquids. It is defined as an inflammation of the lungs due to inhalation of solid or liquid matter. (See AHA *Coding Clinic for ICD-10-CM/PCS,* First Quarter 2017, p. 24.)

CASE STUDIES: EXERCISES IN THE PRACTICAL APPLICATION OF THE CDI REVIEW PROCESS

When the events surrounding the case are pieced together with the documentation in the medical record, the CDI specialist should verify that the documentation reflects to the greatest degree of specificity the conditions present. In this scenario, there are several clues that point to the more specific and more accurate diagnosis of a possible, probable, likely, or suspected aspiration pneumonia as opposed to the more generic diagnosis of pneumonia. The treatment is aimed at Gram-negative coverage, the circumstances of the event reflect a high risk for aspiration, and the CXR report reflects results "suspicious for pneumonia" and point to the right lung as the more specific location.

Due to the anatomy of the bronchus and the more direct line of the right main-stem bronchus, it is more often the right lung that is affected when an aspiration event occurs. The laboratory results reflect an elevated WBC count and elevated neutrophil count. The patient was noted to have a rectal temperature of 101.4°F. All these clinical indicators point to a reasonable cause to query the provider for greater specificity of the condition being treated, as the current documentation reflects "possible pneumonia" and "unknown aspiration."

Respiratory condition specificity

The provider also identifies a second respiratory condition as "acute respiratory distress." The sharp CDI specialist will immediately recognize that the clinical presentation and treatment in this scenario do not correlate to the documented diagnosis. Acute respiratory distress is a term that codes to a sign and symptom code (R06.03) and denotes a very low-acuity diagnosis akin to dyspnea or SOB. Clearly, this scenario depicts a more serious condition as evidenced by endotracheal intubation and mechanical ventilation with high oxygen delivery requirements.

The provider describes the patient as "ventilator dependent" and a pulmonary specialty consult was requested by the attending physician. ABG analysis upon admission further reveals metabolic acidosis, with a high pO_2 of 143 on 100% FiO_2 per AMBU bag assist. Understanding of the P/F ratio is an important concept for the CDI specialist to possess. The P/F ratio is calculated by the formula pO_2/FiO_2 and depicts the true reflection of the pO_2 on room air in the patient who is on supplemental oxygen.

Therefore, this patient, with a pO_2 of 143 while receiving FiO_2 of 100%, has a P/F ratio of 143. A P/F ratio of < 300 is indicative of acute respiratory failure and increased risk for acute respiratory distress syndrome (ARDS). Knowing how to calculate and assess a patient who is receiving supplemental oxygen is an important tool in the CDI specialist's toolkit. It also provides the CDI specialist additional clinical discernment when determining whether a query is justified. A second query to more accurately depict the true clinical picture is again warranted in this case scenario.

Renal condition specificity

As the CDI specialist progresses through this case, yet a third condition presents with clinical indicators and documentation that is discordant, thus more opportunity to achieve greater accuracy in the code assignment. The documentation of acute renal insufficiency may present the prospect of additional specificity when evaluated in concert with the following additional documentation that is present in this case.

First, the patient presented after having been found unresponsive for an unknown period of time and under unknown circumstances for the causative factors. Next, the physical exam and test findings revealed hot and dry skin, a high fever, low urine output, high creatinine kinase (CK) levels, a diagnosis of rhabdomyolysis, high serum creatinine levels with a corresponding low GFR, and urinalysis results of high specific gravity. When these factors are all evaluated within the context of the entire scenario, it would be appropriate to query the provider for additional clarification of the acute renal insufficiency, which is a nonspecific diagnosis with code assignment of low severity.

In comparison, documentation of acute kidney injury (AKI) or AKI with acute tubular necrosis provides a more in-depth and potentially more accurate representation of the true condition and severity associated with the condition.

The Kidney Disease: Improving Global Outcomes (KDIGO) 2012 Clinical Practice Guideline defines AKI as:

- Increase in SCr by ≥ 0.3 mg/dl (≥ 26.5 μmol/l) within 48 hours
- Increase in SCr to ≥ 1.5 times baseline, which is known or presumed to have occurred within the prior 7 days
- Urine volume < 0.5 ml/kg/h for 6 hours

The clinical practice guideline further states that the causes of AKI may include conditions or susceptibilities such as sepsis, critical illness, trauma, dehydration or volume depletion, chronic diseases, advanced age, black race, diabetes mellitus, and female gender. When assessing this case, the presence of several of these factors should guide the CDI specialist in posing a query to the provider.

Infection specificity

A final diagnosis that requires assessment from the CDI specialist is that of the currently documented diagnoses of "acute septic encephalopathy" and "shock." The criteria for sepsis have been studied and reported in the medical literature extensively. The most recent (at the time of this book's writing) was published in the *Journal of the American Medical Association* on February 23, 2016, in a special communication titled *The Third International Consensus Definitions for Sepsis and Septic Shock (Sepsis-3)*. The study proposed that "Sepsis should be defined as life-threatening organ dysfunction caused by a dysregulated host response to infection."

Septic shock is defined by Richard Pinson, MD, FACP, CCS, and Cynthia Tang, RHIA, CCS, in the *2018 CDI Pocket Guide* as "persisting hypotension requiring vasopressors to maintain mean arterial pressure (MAP) > 65 and having a serum lactate level > 2 mmol/L despite adequate volume resuscitation."

Though globally reviewed and debated, the medical community has not universally accepted the new Sepsis-3 guidelines, and a disparity exists among providers as to which set of criteria is used to ascribe a diagnosis of sepsis. There are many practitioners who continue to follow the Sepsis-2 guidelines that were published in 2001. The Surviving Sepsis Campaign, however, officially adopted the definition for Sepsis-3 in March 2017 and in turn payers and auditors often use the Sepsis-3 criteria to evaluate claims.

An important point to appreciate is that Sepsis-3 does not distinguish between the diagnosis of sepsis and the diagnosis of severe sepsis: Sepsis-3 considers that *all* sepsis is severe, thus making the adjective "severe" redundant. The CDI specialist would be wise to have this discussion with physicians to ascertain if there exists a variance within the facility regarding which definition to follow.

Despite this guidance, ICD-10-CM coding remains unchanged with codes for sepsis, unspecified organism (A41.9), Severe sepsis without septic shock (R65.20), and Severe sepsis with septic shock (R65.21). When coding sepsis, the coding professional will code first the underlying infection (or A41.9 if the causative organism cannot be determined). The coding professional will also code the specific acute organ dysfunction, such as acute kidney failure, acute respiratory failure, encephalopathy, disseminated intravascular coagulopathy (DIC), and other such critical conditions.

While these are specific coding guidelines, the knowledgeable CDI specialist will understand and employ these key concepts in their daily practice. When sepsis is due to an artificial device, it is paramount that the cause-and-effect relationship is explicitly documented in the record. An assumption of the correlation cannot be made, and whenever there exists unclear or imprecise documentation, the provider must be queried for clarification. Another important fact the CDI specialist should know is that negative blood cultures do not preclude a diagnosis of sepsis or suspected sepsis; the presence of one or more risk factors, combined with a clear clinical presentation and treatment for the suspected sepsis, is sufficient to diagnose and code sepsis.

CHAPTER 4

With the advent of ICD-10-CM, acute organ dysfunction must be documented as associated with the sepsis; it is not an assumed cause-and-effect relationship. According to the ICD-10-CM *Official Guidelines for Coding and Reporting*, "Acute organ dysfunction must be linked to sepsis in order to assign the severe sepsis code (or provider may document the term severe sepsis). If patient has acute organ dysfunction and sepsis, but no causal relationship is documented, then severe sepsis is not assigned."

Additional conditions to review, consider, and validate

It is fundamental to the CDI process that all diagnoses be validated by a thorough assessment of the clinical indicators appropriate to validate each condition prior to entering the diagnosis into the provisional coding and subsequent DRG assignment. The provider in this scenario has documented metabolic and septic encephalopathy. Septic encephalopathy cannot exist without a diagnosis of sepsis. The documentation of the sepsis, however, is not present in the record and therefore the CDI specialist must query for the infection specificity. The metabolic encephalopathy is clearly documented and can stand up to the scrutiny for the validity of the diagnosis based on the overall clinical scenario and findings.

The diagnosis of acute respiratory insufficiency is addressed through the query process for greater specificity of the respiratory condition. While mechanical ventilation is not a mandatory component of a diagnosis for acute respiratory failure, the clinical scenario presented here supports a diagnosis of much greater severity than "acute respiratory insufficiency," which simply denotes a symptom code equivalent to SOB.

Metabolic acidosis is clearly documented and easily supported in the record with a lactic acid result of 4.8 on admission. The diagnosis of "acute kidney injury" can likely be further specified and is addressed to the provider in a query. The patient was found down for an unknown period of time and was dehydrated as evidenced by the clinical signs outlined in the query, and the probability exists that acute tubular necrosis is a viable and appropriate diagnosis that further illustrates the true SOI.

The definition for shock according to *Dorland's Illustrated Medical Dictionary* is:

> *... a condition of profound hemodynamic and metabolic disturbance characterized by failure of the circulatory system to maintain adequate perfusion of vital organs. It may result from inadequate blood volume (hypovolemic shock), inadequate cardiac function (cardiogenic shock), or inadequate vasomotor tone (neurogenic shock and septic shock).*

CASE STUDIES: EXERCISES IN THE PRACTICAL APPLICATION OF THE CDI REVIEW PROCESS

The evidence for shock is clear in this case scenario, although the type of shock is not clearly documented. Shock can be delineated as hypovolemic, cardiovascular, neurogenic, septic, toxic, anaphylactic, post-procedural, and other forms of shock. A query for the type of shock is warranted and included in the infection specificity query to the provider.

While this case presents many prospects for the CDI specialist to glean further specificity of the documentation in the medical record, it is important to remain cognizant of the intent of the query and need for greater clarification. Not each and every diagnosis may need to be queried. Yet in some cases, there is greater need to clarify multiple diagnoses in order to maintain and ensure the integrity of the final record. All conditions that are integral to the integrity of the record should be critically analyzed, and a determination should be made by the CDI specialist as to when a query is appropriate and necessary.

The CDI specialist should maintain an awareness of the tendency to "over query" when a diagnosis is not integral to the overall integrity and clinical truth reflected in the final coded record. Conversely, when the record contains gaps in documentation that are relevant to reflecting the true SOI, ROM, and intensity of the services rendered, the CDI specialist should indeed query and support that effort with education and interaction with the care providers.

References for sepsis

The *ICD-10 Official Guidelines for Coding and Reporting* contain the following definitions of several common terms related to sepsis:

- Bacteremia: The presence of bacteria in the blood without a systemic disease
- SIRS: Noninfectious systemic response to trauma, burns, or other insults
- Sepsis: Systemic inflammatory response syndrome due to infectious process without acute organ dysfunction
- Severe sepsis: Systemic inflammatory response syndrome due to infectious process with acute organ dysfunction
- Severe sepsis with septic shock: Shock associated with overwhelming infection, usually infection with Gram-negative bacteria, although it may be produced by other bacteria, viruses, fungi, or protozoa

---

Source: *ICD-10 Official Guidelines for Coding and Reporting.*

CHAPTER 4

Case Study: Neoplastic Disease

Case study: Neoplastic disease

History of present illness: An 86-year-old male presented to the ED with a chief complaint of worsening hoarseness, cough, and abdominal pain. He describes his abdominal pain as feeling "bloated" and hard to the touch. Upon further questioning, he admits that he has been having abdominal pain on and off for more than six months. He describes his hoarseness as chronic but getting worse. He denies nausea, vomiting, diarrhea, constipation, and change in bowel patterns. Patient states he has no appetite and cannot eat much anyway due to his constant feeling of "fullness." Admits to a 35-pound weight loss in the past year. I suspect this is due to underlying malignancy.

Past medical history: The patient has a past medical history of CAD status post CABG, fluorodeoxyglucose avid (FDG-avid) lung nodule, pneumonia, chronic hoarseness, benign prostatic hyperplasia, and restless leg syndrome. He was diagnosed two years ago with a pulmonary nodule which was discovered incidentally while he was being treated for pneumonia. A repeat CT scan at the time showed the pneumonia resolving, but a right upper lobe (RUL) pulmonary nodule was determined to be positive for FDG uptake and 1.5 cm in size. He subsequently underwent a laryngoscopy that showed bilateral vocal cord neoplasms but he refused further workup at the time. It should be noted the patient has a 60-pack-per-year tobacco use and chronic hoarseness.

Home medications: NKDA, baby Aspirin once daily, Tamsulosin 0.4 mg daily, Gabapentin 300 mg TID

Physical exam:

- **General:** Alert and oriented ×3. Cooperative and in obvious discomfort.
- **Heart:** HR regular, no murmurs, gallops, or rub.
- **Lungs:** Lungs bilaterally clear to auscultation anteriorly and posteriorly.
- **Integumentary:** Skin is warm, dry, poor skin turgor. No lymphadenopathy noted.
- **Gastrointestinal:** Normal bowel sounds, generally distended abdomen with massive hepatomegaly felt on examination. Right upper and middle quadrant vascular markings evident. However, no signs for ascites. Patient complained of extreme discomfort on deep palpation in the epigastric and right lower quadrant regions.
- **Vital signs:** BP 128/88; HR 90; RR 19; temperature 98.2°F; FiO_2 saturation 94% on room air; BMI 21.

CASE STUDIES: EXERCISES IN THE PRACTICAL APPLICATION OF THE CDI REVIEW PROCESS

Treatment: Pain control, CT thorax and abdomen, liver ultrasound, dietary consult, gentle hydration, and will order IV if unable to tolerate fluids orally.

Clinical findings

Radiology: CT of thorax and abdomen suspicious for lesions in liver. Stable RUL nodule noted to be similar in size as previous study.

Liver ultrasound: Patient declined any further studies or treatment.

Registered dietitian notes: Patient with bilateral vocal cord neoplasms and unintentional weight loss of 35 pounds in the past year. He agrees to supplemental calorie intake. Counseled to eat small portions in more frequent meals as tolerated.

LABORATORY FINDINGS

	Day 3	Day 2	Day 1
Alpha-fetoprotein			High
WBC	6.8	6.9	7.2
Hgb	11.0 (L)	11.4 (L)	11.0 (L)
Hct	34.6 (L)	34.6 (L)	34.2 (L)
Platelets	183	185	178
Neutrophils	5.0	4.9	5.0
Na+	136	135	135
K+	4.3	4.2	4.2
CL−	107	104	104
CO_2	19 (L)	20 (L)	19 (L)
Blood glucose	86	92	78
BUN	22	46 (H)	56 (H)

CHAPTER 4

	Day 3	Day 2	Day 1
Creatinine	1.02	1.49 (H)	1.55 (H)
GFR	91	45 (L)	43 (L)
Albumin	3.0 (L)	2.5 (L)	2.6 (L)
Alkaline phosphatase	310 (H)	339 (H)	337 (H)
Bilirubin, total	1.2 (H)	1.2 (H)	1.6 (H)
ALT	58 (H)	57 (H)	58 (H)
AST	117 (H)	122 (H)	119 (H)
Lactic acid			2.9 (H)

Impression

1. GI consulted for evaluation of hepatomegaly in 86-year-old male with vocal cord neoplasm and FDG-avid lung nodule

2. The etiology of the massive hepatomegaly is highly suspicious for infiltrative metastatic cancer

3. Anion gap acidosis

4. Elevated renal indexes

5. Elevated liver indexes

6. Loss of appetite, chronic disease

NOTES

QUERY: NEOPLASM

Clinical indicators

1. "... laryngoscopy which showed bilateral vocal cord neoplasms," per Dr. Attending H&P 2/11/2017

2. "The etiology of the massive hepatomegaly is highly suspicious for infiltrative metastatic cancer," per Dr. Attending H&P 2/11/2017

3. "CT of thorax and abdomen suspicious for lesions in liver," per consult note GI 2/12/17

4. "right upper lobe pulmonary nodule was determined to be positive for FDG uptake and 1.5 cm in size," per Dr. Attending progress note 2/12/2017

Request for clarification: Malignancy

Dr. Attending,

The medical record reflects a diagnosis of malignancy. Can you please clarify the known or suspected primary site of the malignancy and the known or suspected sites of any metastases?

Thank you,
CDI Specialist, contact information

CHAPTER 4

Options for response

- Primary site of malignancy _____
- Metastatic site(s) of malignancy _____
- Clinically undetermined primary site of malignancy
- Clinically undetermined presence of secondary or metastatic site(s) of malignancy
- Other, please specify

CASE STUDIES: EXERCISES IN THE PRACTICAL APPLICATION OF THE CDI REVIEW PROCESS

QUERY: NUTRITION

Clinical indicators

1. "Admits to a 35-pound weight loss in the past year. I suspect this is due to underlying malignancy," per Dr. Attending H&P 2/11/2017

2. ". . . dietary consult . . ." per treatment plan Dr. Attending H&P 2/11/2017

3. BMI 21 per electronic health record

4. "He agrees to supplemental calorie intake," per registered dietitian notes 2/12/2017

Request for clarification: Nutritional status

Dr. Attending,

Can the nutritional status of this patient be further specified? If yes, please note below.

Thank you,
CDI specialist, contact information

CHAPTER 4

Options for response

- No nutrition-related diagnosis
- No malnutrition
- Mild/first-degree malnutrition
- Moderate/second-degree malnutrition
- Severe/third-degree malnutrition
- Other nutritional diagnosis _____
- Unable to determine

QUERY: RENAL CONDITION

Clinical indicators

1. "Elevated renal indexes," per impression Dr. Attending H&P 2/11/2017

2. "Gentle hydration and will order IV if unable to tolerate fluids orally," per treatment plan Dr. Attending H&P 2/11/2017

3. Laboratory findings:

	Day 3	Day 2	Day 1
BUN	22	46 (H)	56 (H)
Creatinine	1.02	1.49 (H)	1.55 (H)
GFR	91	45 (L)	43 (L)

Request for clarification: Renal condition

Dr. Attending,

Please further clarify the diagnosis of "elevated renal indexes" and etiology if known.

Thank you,

CDI Specialist, contact information

CHAPTER 4

Options for response

- Acute renal insufficiency
- Acute kidney injury
    - With tubular necrosis
    - With cortical necrosis
- Chronic kidney disease
    - CKD stage 1
    - CKD stage 2 (mild)
    - CKD stage 3 (moderate)
- Underlying cause
    - Dehydration
- Other _____
- Unable to determine _____

CASE STUDIES: EXERCISES IN THE PRACTICAL APPLICATION OF THE CDI REVIEW PROCESS

Case study discussion

Once again, the seasoned CDI specialist who encounters a case scenario as described in this one will be challenged to critically analyze several aspects of the case, multiple concurrent conditions, as well as an often rapidly evolving clinical picture. Some of the elements of the review are obvious, and the CDI specialist can easily focus on those diagnoses that need further clarification. When faced with multiple body systems that are affected, however, a sound clinical foundation is essential to a thorough and complete review. Likewise, a deep fundamental knowledge of pathophysiology and acute care medicine will serve the CDI specialist well in a complex review such as this.

As the CDI specialist reviews the information presented in this case, there are key factors that should stand out to prompt the investigative process that is central to an expert CDI review. This scenario starts with a patient who has preexisting testing that points to an increased likelihood for malignancy. Similar to the previous case scenario, as the CDI specialist examines the records, there are several questions that should surface and require greater inspection by the CDI specialist.

Overview

A good place to begin in this scenario is a thoughtful evaluation of the patient's history of the incidental finding of a pulmonary nodule two years ago while being treated for pneumonia. A subsequent workup at that time revealed the right upper lobe to be positive for a FDG-avid nodule. While that finding may or may not be definitive for a diagnosis of malignancy, the suspicion for such is heightened.

When an astute CDI specialist assesses this finding in association with the current documentation of "unintentional weight loss," "loss of appetite," "60-pack-per-year tobacco use and chronic hoarseness" which the patient describes as worsening, and a "laryngoscopy which showed bilateral vocal cord neoplasms," they should correlate these findings and begin to investigate the conditions and the possibility that they may be related. The CDI specialist should conduct the record review while mindful of the possible interrelatedness of these conditions while searching for clues.

Malignancy clarification and specificity

Coding for neoplasms and metastases is very specific, and the CDI specialist should familiarize him- or herself with the idiosyncrasies of coding and documentation of neoplasms as the primary or the metastatic site. When the treatment and the objective of the admission are to treat the primary malignancy, the primary malignancy should be coded as the principal diagnosis. The exception to this rule is when a patient admission/encounter is solely for the administration of chemotherapy, immunotherapy, or radiation therapy. In that case, assign the appropriate Z51 code as the principal diagnosis and the diagnosis or problem for which the service is being performed as a secondary diagnosis.

There are several guidelines that govern the coding of neoplasms and interrelated conditions. A comprehensive understanding of these guidelines is suggested for every CDI specialist. Knowing and understanding these guidelines empowers the CDI specialist to know when to ask for greater clarification in the medical record and under what circumstances that clarification will affect and influence coding.

This scenario reflects a history of bilateral vocal cord neoplasms for which no treatment has been administered since the diagnosis two years prior to this encounter for care. It is reasonable to query the provider for any suspected metastases given the patient has not sought any treatment since the original diagnosis and there are symptoms present that suggest additional organ or tissue involvement outside the vocal cords. Those symptoms include definitive laryngoscopy findings for bilateral vocal cord neoplasms, "massive hepatomegaly (that) is highly suspicious for infiltrative metastatic cancer," positive CT of the abdomen findings that are "suspicious for lesions in the liver," and an unintended weight loss of 35 pounds over one year, suspected "due to underlying malignancy."

Nutritional clarification and specificity

It is important to note that although this patient has a current BMI of 21, that does not preclude a diagnosis of malnutrition to some degree. This patient has evidence of a chronic, debilitating, and life-threatening disease. He has experienced an unintentional 35-pound weight loss over the past year, admits to loss of appetite, has a life-threatening debilitative illness, and demonstrates significant risk for malnutrition based on the fact that his abdominal discomfort, bloating, and tightness do not permit him to take in meals sufficient to meet his caloric requirement.

Given these factors, it is reasonable and appropriate for the CDI specialist to query the physician for a more specific diagnosis. Malnutrition is a diagnosis that is often underdiagnosed in the acute care population and is described as "a major contributor to increased morbidity and mortality, decreased function and quality of life, increased frequency and length of hospital stay, and higher healthcare costs." It reflects an increased SOI and ROM and should be clarified in the medical record whenever the clinical criteria support the additional specificity of the diagnosis. Although the albumen level is low at 2.5 (normal is 3.5–5.0 gm/dL), factors that influence albumin levels and prealbumin levels extend far beyond malnutrition. Therefore, these values are not considered indicative of malnutrition.

CASE STUDIES: EXERCISES IN THE PRACTICAL APPLICATION OF THE CDI REVIEW PROCESS

The World Health Organization defines malnutrition as "deficiencies, excesses, or imbalances in a person's intake of energy and/or nutrients." The term "malnutrition" addresses three broad groups of conditions:

- Undernutrition, which includes wasting (low weight for height), stunting (low height for age), and underweight (low weight for age)

- Micronutrient-related malnutrition, which includes micronutrient deficiencies (a lack of important vitamins and minerals) or micronutrient excess

- Overweight, obesity, and diet-related noncommunicable diseases (such as heart disease, stroke, diabetes, and some cancers)

In a highly developed country such as the United States, micronutrient malnutrition is more common in the low-income, elderly, or chronically ill patient populations. As such, it is not uncommon to observe patients who have been adequately nourished throughout their lifespan suddenly become undernourished when faced with chronic debilitating disease and subsequent loss of appetite. The CDI specialist should remain alert when reviewing records of this high-risk population to ensure that complete, concise, and consistent documentation of this comorbid condition is appropriately captured in the documentation, therefore reflecting the true SOI and ROM.

Renal condition clarification and specificity

It is not surprising that this patient exhibits signs of renal dysfunction, given his loss of appetite and inability to ingest fluids and food due to the abdominal discomfort and tightness. A query for the specificity of the renal dysfunction is clearly indicated, as the physician's documentation of "elevated renal indexes" simply notates (and codes to) abnormal lab findings (R79.9). The additional specificity and documentation of AKI will more accurately reflect the treatment for hydration and possible intravenous fluid administration as indicated by the provider in the plan of treatment.

In the setting of a patient who has a chronic and life-threatening condition coupled with the nutritional compromise, the additional complication of renal dysfunction makes matters much worse when the entire scenario is assessed. The CDI specialist should investigate these additional conditions and the added specificity level even when a patient may be considered for hospice or have signed a "Do not resuscitate" (DNR) order. Though that is not the case here, the integrity of the medical record that reflects the truest and purest form of diagnosis specificity should be the goal of every CDI specialist.

CHAPTER 4

Additional considerations

When a provider asks why it's important to note malnutrition in a patient who's clearly dying anyway, the CDI specialist needs to understand that the critical nature of all the patient's conditions written in their medical record should entirely reflect *why* that patient is in the end stage of life and is "clearly dying." After all, healthy patients should not die. It is only the sickest of patients, with the highest scoring of SOI/ROM scores, who should be dying.

Often, I teach that when documentation of SOI and ROM are low, yet the patient succumbs to death, only one of two scenarios can be at play. Either the documentation of the patient's condition is poor and inadequate, or the medical care administered to the patient is poor and inadequate. When I ask the physician which of those scenarios is the accurate picture of the case, I can guarantee you the response is never "the care administered to the patient was poor and inadequate."

I rest my case. Documentation of the greatest specificity for each and every diagnosis relevant to the patient's encounter for care is vital to the integrity of the final coded medical record. It accurately reflects the SOI, the ROM, the intensity of the resources used to care for the patient, and the complexity of the entire clinical scenario, reflective of the physician's medical decision-making skills and expert knowledge.

REFERENCES

3M. (n.d.). 3M Codefinder.

Acute Kidney Injury (AKI). (n.d.). Retrieved July 13, 2018, from *https://kdigo.org/guidelines/acute-kidney-injury/*.

Almuhaideb, A., Papathanasiou, N., & Bomanji, J. (2011). ^{18}F-FDG PET/CT Imaging In Oncology. *Annals of Saudi Medicine, 31*(1), 3–13. http://doi.org/10.4103/0256-4947.75771.

The American Hospital Association. (1988). *Coding Clinic for ICD-9-CM, third quarter*, 11. Retrieved July 14, 2018.

The American Hospital Association. (2017). *Coding Clinic for ICD-10-CM, first quarter*, 24. Retrieved July 14, 2018.

Archibald, L. (2018, June 14). Note from the ACDIS Editor: ACDIS resources on malnutrition. *CDI Strategies*, vol. 12:27.

The Association of Clinical Documentation Improvement Specialists. (2009). *Cut through the confusion of altered mental status* (Publication). Middleton, MA: HCPro.

The Association of Clinical Documentation Improvement Specialists. (2018, April 19). ACDIS update: ACDIS poll reveals members' top 10 queried diagnoses. *CDI Strategies*, vol. 12:16.

Centers for Disease Control and Prevention. (2017, April 26). Retrieved July 5, 2018, from *https://www.cdc.gov/*.

Centers for Medicare and Medicaid Services, & National Center for Health Statistics. (2018). *ICD-10-CM Official Guidelines for Coding and Reporting.*

CASE STUDIES: EXERCISES IN THE PRACTICAL APPLICATION OF THE CDI REVIEW PROCESS

Clinical Documentation Improvement Desk Reference - ICD-10-CM & Procedure Coding 2018. (2017). Optuminsight.

Dorland, W. A. (2012). *Dorland's illustrated medical dictionary.* Philadelphia, PA: Saunders/Elsevier.

Pinson, R. D., & Tang, C. L. (2017). *2018 CDI Pocket Guide.* Middleton, MA: HCPro.

Singer, M., Deutschman, C. S., & Seymour, C. W., et. al. (2016). The Third International Consensus Definitions for Sepsis and Septic Shock (Sepsis-3). *The Journal of the American Medical Association, 315*(8), 801-810. Retrieved July 13, 2018, from *https://jamanetwork.com/.*

Straight A Nursing Student. (n.d.). Retrieved July 13, 2018, from *www.straightanursingstudent.com/.*

Teasdale, G., & Jennett, B. (1974). Trauma Scoring: Glasgow Coma Score. Retrieved July 14, 2018, from *www.trauma.org/archive/scores/gcs.html.*

Vassalotti, J. A., Centor, R., Turner, B. J., Greer, R. C., Choi, M., & Sequist, T. D. (2016). Practical Approach to Detection and Management of Chronic Kidney Disease for the Primary Care Clinician. *The American Journal of Medicine, 129*(2), 153–162. doi:10.1016/j.amjmed.2015.08.025

White, J. V., Guenter, P., Jensen, G., Malone, A., & Schofield, M. (2012). Consensus Statement of the Academy of Nutrition and Dietetics/American Society for Parenteral and Enteral Nutrition: Characteristics Recommended for the Identification and Documentation of Adult Malnutrition (Undernutrition). *Journal of the Academy of Nutrition and Dietetics,* 112(5), 730–738. doi:10.1016/j.jand.2012.03.012.

CHAPTER 5

Leading and Managing a CDI Program

CDI Program Evolution

The clinical documentation improvement (CDI) world has undergone radical change since the first programs began about two decades ago. Many CDI programs were formed under the umbrella of case management, quality assurance programs, business and revenue, or the health information management (HIM) department. The purpose of the CDI specialist was often unclear and enmeshed with goals of the department in which they were housed. CDI daily duties often aligned more to core measure reviews, managing length of stay (LOS), or assigning a Diagnosis-Related Group (DRG) with optimal capture of complications or comorbid conditions (CC) and major CCs (MCC).

Since these beginnings, however, the models of CDI have evolved and become more focused on documentation integrity as a whole. Many programs remain connected to the case management, quality, or revenue cycle departments and work very well in those models. More frequently, however, CDI programs are either aligned with the HIM department or exist as a separate standalone department. According to the 2017 CDI Salary Survey from the Association of Clinical Documentation Improvement Specialists (ACDIS), 34.77% of CDI programs report to the HIM department, 19.88% function as standalone departments, 11.62% report to the chief financial officer, 11.24% report to case management, 8.26% report to quality, and 2.5% report to the chief medical officer.

Whatever the organizational structure may be, however, it is evident that CDI has a separate and distinct function that is essential to the organization. CDI touches numerous points in the operation of the organization; revenue cycle, business office, denials management, establishment of the "working DRG" and subsequent geometric mean LOS (GMLOS) for proper case management and discharge planning, and

CHAPTER 5

identification of concurrent quality measures that may adversely affect patient outcomes. CDI professionals are key to identifying the greatest specificity necessary in the concurrent medical record to accurately reflect the true clinical condition, severity of illness, risk of mortality, and intensity of resources expended during the encounter to care for the patient. This effect transfers over to the final coded and billed medical record, but CDI program leadership needs to know how to adequately measure this widespread effect.

CDI Program Leadership

The development and management of an effective and impactful CDI program requires thoughtful planning, execution, and leadership from the organization's key stakeholders. ACDIS published a white paper in 2017 that addresses many of the challenges CDI programs face. According to the paper, "this transformation begins with effective leadership—which is not the same thing as management. Leadership has far less to do with authority and much more to do with setting a vision, mission, and strategy toward specific goals."

Leaders operate more from a high-level perspective of overall mission and vision. Managers more closely align with the day-to-day operational perspective, with great attention to process and details. Each role is vital to the success and impact of the program; developing a team of individual CDI professionals that are astute, highly competent, and respected members of the multidisciplinary care team is essential to program success and impact.

Leaders often possess certain attributes and qualities that foster employee commitment and loyalty. According to an article in *Forbes Magazine*, the following attributes are the eight essential qualities that define great leadership.

1. Sincerity

2. Integrity

3. Great communication skills

4. Loyalty

5. Decisiveness

6. Managerial competence

7. Empowerment

8. Charisma

"Every one of these qualities is absolutely essential to great leadership. Without them, leaders cannot live up to their full potential. As a result, their employees will never perform as well as they can either. Because of this, organizations must learn the best ways to identify and also to develop these necessary traits in existing and emerging leaders," the article says. As we move forward in developing great CDI programs, we must maintain the awareness that developing great leaders for these programs is essential to success.

Daniel M. Cable describes leadership in his book *Alive at Work* as, "when you're a leader—no matter how long you've been in your role or how hard the journey was to get there—you are merely overhead unless you're bringing out the best in your employees. Unfortunately, many leaders lose sight of this." Cable goes on to say that "by focusing too much on control and end goals, and not enough on their people, leaders are making it more difficult to achieve their own desired outcomes."

It's wise to keep that in mind when developing metrics to measure performance and impact of the CDI program and the individual CDI team members. Data collection without the mind-set of "servant-leadership" for the core persons who drive that performance and impact is misguided at best and likely destructive to the core values of the mission.

CDI Program Management

Given the relatively recent onset of CDI programs, it's not surprising that there is a shortage of qualified CDI specialists. As a result, many programs train and educate their own CDI specialists from within the organization, as discussed in Chapter 1. Others may recruit CDI specialists from regional or national consortiums. Whatever the approach, the CDI manager must ensure the competency and effectiveness of each CDI specialist.

The CDI manager is often tasked with ensuring an effective CDI process inclusive of:

- Prioritization of reviews

- Distribution of reviews

CHAPTER 5

- Provisional coding
- Discharge planning
- Query submission
- Quality of care metrics

Let's look at each of these tasks in turn.

Prioritization of reviews

Prioritization of reviews begins with defining the population of cases to be reviewed. This should align closely with the mission of the CDI program. If the mission is largely revenue driven, the most populous payer populations may be a primary filter in determining which cases the CDI specialists review. This was often the case in the beginning stages of CDI program development. Most programs, however, have evolved to include all payers as a matter of avoiding even remotely looking like the program is unfairly focusing on high-volume payers.

If the mission more closely aligns with HIM and coding goals, then the payer is often an irrelevant factor. Rather, identification of often under-documented diagnoses and conditions may be more appropriate factors to consider when determining which cases to review.

A CDI program that is quality driven has optics that are keenly sensitive to hospital-acquired conditions (HAC), patient safety indicators (PSI), mortality associated data, and other quality data reported publicly. No matter the focus of the program, it is essential that a well-defined process is established to determine workflow and impact for the organization in alignment with the CDI program mission.

Regardless of the program's focus, the development of robust and complex, artificial intelligence–based systems in the field of CDI has presented CDI specialists with opportunities to impact the integrity of the medical record in more efficient ways than ever before. The days of paper-based CDI reviews are becoming almost nonexistent in giving way to the more efficient Health Level Seven International (HL7)–driven interface between the electronic health record (EHR) and the CDI review platform.

> **DID YOU KNOW?**
>
> For those who don't know, an HL7, according to *TechTarget*, is "a set of standards, formats and definitions for exchanging and developing electronic health records (EHRs). HL7 standards, developed and promulgated by the healthcare IT standard-setting authority HL7 International, are the de facto standards in healthcare IT, though some HL7 users have called on Congress to create stronger legal interoperability standards for the healthcare IT industry."

Distribution of reviews

Daily workflow process can be distributed in a number of ways, and many organizations take an approach that best fits the unique factors that influence the organization. Some assignments may be location-based. While one CDI specialist is assigned to all the units in a specific wing or location of the hospital, a second CDI specialist may be assigned to all the units in a neighboring wing or tower. This approach often works well in large facilities where much time is wasted in traversing across the entire facility campus.

Conversely, with the introduction of remotely based CDI reviews, physical location is neutralized as a factor. Another approach to assignments is based on service line and allocating specific service lines to specific CDI specialists. For example, a CDI specialist with a strong foundation in cardiovascular surgical nursing may be assigned the cardiovascular surgery service line, as well as cardiology or even critical care medicine. This approach also affords CDI specialists the time and focus to get to know the physicians in their service line personally, which may in turn improve query response rates and physician buy-in. This is a major contributing factor as to why a CDI program may choose to structure itself based on service lines.

The development of CDI software programs that utilize artificial intelligence to prescreen the medical record has changed the landscape of both identification of records that need review and also allocation of those identified cases. Optimizing CDI specialist resources through these sophisticated software platforms serves to more efficiently allocate the precious resource of the highly skilled CDI specialist.

CHAPTER 5

> **DISCUSSION POINT**
>
> Despite many advances in the area of EHR and CDI software, many CDI programs still use a hybrid paper and electronic medical record. In fact, according to the 2018 CDI Week Industry Survey from ACDIS, 24.82% of respondents still had hybrid records.
>
> This situation often opens up quite the conundrum for reporting purposes and CDI program leaders should be prepared to work with their information technology (IT) department at their organization to access the best possible data and sort that data accurately across the two systems. Alternatively, many CDI program leaders develop homegrown tools using spreadsheets to manually track and report their program's progress.

Provisional coding

Provisional coding during the concurrent CDI review process serves to enable case management and utilization management resources more effectively for discharge planning. An accurate and timely provisional or working DRG is an invaluable resource to drive appropriate discharge planning. While many CDI specialists who come from a clinical background may tell you, "I don't know much about coding. It's complicated and I don't know all the sequencing rules," the seasoned CDI specialist is actually quite skilled in the area of coding.

Many CDI specialists come from a purely coding background, while others who have a purely clinical background seek additional education in the coding realm and have attained certification in the field of coding. Regardless of the foundational background, the coding software available empowers all CDI specialists to gain knowledge and expertise in coding through daily learning and building of a solid understanding of key coding concepts.

Query development is a cornerstone of the CDI process. Knowing when to query, how to query, whom to query, and the impact of the query to the final coded medical record is an aptitude CDI specialists learn over time. Many factors enter into play when a CDI specialist is faced with a potential opportunity to glean additional specificity or granularity in the medical record. The mission of the specific CDI program will factor in. The culture of the organization will serve as an additional factor. Additionally, the specific medical record platform used in the organization impacts the communication between CDI specialists and providers and is yet another factor in the query process. Therefore, a keen awareness of these elements will serve the CDI specialist well in determining query development opportunities and submission.

LEADING AND MANAGING A CDI PROGRAM

When the mission of the CDI program has an emphasis on quality of care metrics and publicly reported data, CDI specialists must also possess a thorough understanding of the nuances and intricacies of the Agency for Healthcare Research and Quality (AHRQ) data.

> **DID YOU KNOW?**
>
> The data collected by the AHRQ have historically been available on the National Guidelines Clearinghouse and the National Quality Measures Clearinghouse. As of July 16, 2018, however, both Clearinghouses have been defunded and shut down.
>
> The Emergency Care Research Institute (ECRI) plans to take over the National Guidelines Clearinghouse in the near future, though. CDI professionals should be aware of any developments thereof, especially if their CDI program has a quality-focused mission statement.

Some CDI programs choose to stratify the CDI specialists into areas of expertise, with some members of the team having quality-focused assignments while others may have a more HIM and coding focus. Each approach is compelling on its own accord. It's important to note that an overly broad approach and focus of the CDI reviews may lead to dilution of the CDI program mission. The CDI manager and leadership should always maintain the true intent of the program and align tasks accordingly to support that mission.

CDI specialist development

A CDI program that invests time, energy, and resources into the professional development of its CDI specialists will find that the return on that investment is invaluable. The CDI specialist who has been firmly grounded in the CDI process will return that investment multifold. A CDI specialist who has been supported in developing a professional alliance with physician providers, who has been taught to work in concert with the coding professional, and who has been empowered to use his or her skills and expertise to further the mission of the CDI program is a treasured asset to the organization.

We all likely agree that the above-described CDI specialist is a valuable member of the CDI team. You may want to refer back to Chapter 1 to review the more detailed specifics of CDI specialist development and education. The point I will add here is that continued success of the program is dependent upon continued development of the CDI specialist. Education, training, and skill set development is a dynamic process and should always be in forward momentum.

Many programs employ continuing education on an as-needed basis for their CDI professionals, offering both one-on-one and group educational sessions. Other programs set a more structured cadence for ongoing education, taking a day out of each month for dedicated education. Increasingly, CDI programs have taken advantage of their facility's shared server to store various educational tools, PowerPoints, and even recorded webinars for quick reference by the CDI specialists.

Regardless of the specific tactics employed, remember that a CDI program that remains satisfied with the initial CDI training is likely to become stagnant. The exciting and challenging aspect of CDI is that it is a profession that is rapidly morphing into new and unique areas that positively impact the landscape of healthcare across many continuums. We are a vibrant and unique population of healthcare professionals who are on the leading edge of regulatory initiatives as well as healthcare research for improved patient care through a more precise statistical compilation of diseases. The imprint we can leave for the healthcare profession is a frontier not yet fully realized.

Measurement of CDI program goals

A CDI program should be measured against performance metrics that are aligned with its established mission statement and goals. Regular reporting, through a dashboard designed to assess, measure, and track performance, is an approach many organizations successfully employ. The ability to filter metrics reflective of program performance is fundamental to adjusting the data to address the particular focus and investment of the various departments within the organization.

Some organizations may have the means and desire to acquire, either through a vendor or consulting company, preformatted software designed to reflect the key metrics of the CDI program. Other organizations may choose to develop a customized dashboard in-house through either the facility's IT department or by using a spreadsheet. While either approach is reasonable depending on the funding available for CDI program efforts, the crucial elements of the CDI program impact and performance should be included to reflect the true effect for the organization.

LEADING AND MANAGING A CDI PROGRAM

Measuring CDI program impact is multifaceted and requires a fundamental understanding of the true intent of the program. Various stakeholders may assess the CDI program from narrowly focused metrics driven from their unique perspective. Therefore, it's imperative that CDI leadership drive the conversation to include all the touch points that CDI impacts. These touch points may encompass many areas such as:

- Severity of illness (SOI) and risk of mortality (ROM)
- Case-mix index (CMI)
- CDI review rates
- CDI query rates
- Physician query response rates
- Physician query response impact
- Top DRGs by volume
- Financial impact

The Big Data, the Little Data, and the "Intangible" Data

The big data review of the CDI program often is the set of metrics reported to senior leadership for the organization. It often takes the most key performance metrics and reports in a monthly or quarterly trending account. Year-over-year data can be analyzed and trended to drive program initiatives. A report that is succinct and significant to the mission of the CDI program and supportive of the organization's mission is key to ensure the focus of the "big data" is relevant to the audience of senior leadership.

Another aspect of CDI program surveillance is drilling into the "little data." The little data is more reflective of the daily and weekly CDI process. CDI workflow processes may be monitored using this data. Obstacles for success of the CDI program may be identified at this level of data analysis. Software issues that affect CDI productivity performance may be identified and thus CDI management can propel a timely and acceptable resolution to the problem. The query process may prove to be time intensive when software programs do not facilitate seamless transfer of queries to and from the provider. CDI managers who are intimately aware of the CDI workflow of the team will better serve the program through

CHAPTER 5

active engagement in driving initiatives designed to remove barriers to successful performance and program outcomes.

The intangible data is much subtler, and it may prove more difficult to assign absolute values to this data. By the intangible data, I mean the impact CDI has on the avoidance of risk for:

- Denials
- Errors in code assignment
- Inaccurate quality metrics
- Incorrect publicly reported data, both for the organization and the providers

Avoidance and reduction of risk are hard to assign specific financial figures. It is difficult to financially demonstrate the return on investment (ROI) for the CDI program. That is sometimes a challenging conversation to have with the executive chief financial officer (CFO) or chief executive officer (CEO) in an organization. Yet, it is critical that the impact of CDI be conveyed accurately and effectively to this audience. Communication of the intangible data to the C-suite team can be challenging at best and often frustrating. No single approach or verbiage will work in every situation. The astute CDI leader, however, will understand what uniquely matters to the CFO, what matters to the CEO, and what matters to the chief medical officer (CMO). Each of these chiefs may view the value of the CDI program in a slightly different manner that most closely aligns with their scope of accountability. Therefore, it is crucial that the CDI leadership conveys the appropriate message to the appropriate audience, in an appropriate and impactful format and at a suitable time for optimal effect.

When delivering a message to the CFO, it's important to understand his or her perspective and which data matters to them specifically. If the CMI has dropped in a given time period, the CFO might ascribe that drop to improper coding practices. A root cause analysis by expert CDI leadership, however, can address these variances with poise and proficiency, explaining that a decrease in surgical volume in a service line of especially high relative weighting (such as cardiovascular surgery) may be the more accurate cause of the CMI variance. When presented alongside reports that demonstrate coding accuracy scores reflective of low error rates, this data can further serve to explain the various factors that affect the CMI fluctuations.

When addressing the CEO who is concerned about dropping ratings in the hospital's publicly reported *HealthGrades* scores, it's important that the CDI leadership understand what factors determine those scores.

LEADING AND MANAGING A CDI PROGRAM

For example, knowledge of the factors that drive the *HealthGrades* Patient Safety Excellence Award will empower the CDI manager to address issues that originate in poor documentation practices versus issues that arise from poor physician engagement with responding to queries that are intended to improve the subpar documentation performance. Additional knowledge of the core set of patient safety indicators and understanding of Medicare Provider and Analysis Review (MedPAR) data will further serve the CDI leader to appropriately address quality concerns the CEO may hold for the organization.

The CMO may embrace metrics surrounding avoidance of excess days in the hospital, aligning with key utilization management initiatives and risk avoidance of adverse events that could result from prolonged hospital stays. Demonstration of the correlation between accurate and complete documentation of all relevant conditions and the accurate DRG assignment with the accurate GMLOS can serve to further CDI program physician engagement. When physician engagement with query response is poor, and the correlation of the lost opportunities for documentation specificity are tied to that poor response rate, then it can be quite advantageous for the CDI leader to "connect the dots" from poor documentation practices and excessive LOS, because the DRG may not accurately reflect the true SOI and ROM the patient possesses.

While it may be easy to discuss and recommend data collection and surveillance, it is much more difficult to make that collection a reality. The January/February 2018 edition of ACDIS' *CDI Journal* includes a fascinating article entitled *Case Study: CDI informaticist eases data woes*. You may ask "What exactly is a CDI informaticist?" While not a common role found in CDI programs, those CDI programs that do employ this role often find this resource to be invaluable.

A CDI informaticist is skilled in many areas, including positive communication skills, IT, data analytics, and the healthcare environment. A CDI informaticist that possesses a comprehensive knowledge of the scope of the CDI program can effectively pull data together. The data can in turn serve to highlight areas of opportunity to strengthen the program as well as underscore areas of excellence. Reporting out metrics to key stakeholders may include senior executive leadership, medical staff leadership and its individual members, and CDI leaders and the individual CDI specialists. Reporting the metrics is one aspect, but a methodical analysis of the data—what it tells us and what it doesn't tell us—is more to the point of the matter. An informaticist can add that element of proficiency that leadership can capitalize on to propel the CDI program and its impact to even greater gains for the organization.

CHAPTER 5

Conclusion

A successful CDI program should begin with a clear vision and mission statement that succinctly and wholly describes that vision and intent. The mission of the program often encompasses a wide range of impactful measures across the organization such as quality, utilization management, financial, patient care, public profiling, and resource allocation. Ultimately, the CDI program of today is multifaceted and integral to the overall organizational well-being.

Additionally, the CDI specialist is a vibrant and vital member of the healthcare team, adding value in numerous ways previously mentioned at numerous points throughout this book. While the CDI specialist often leaves an imprint that may segue into many other elements of the total patient encounter, the key responsibility for the CDI specialist remains to ensure the integrity of the medical record. This is accomplished through a thoughtful and critical analysis of the clinical factors, treatments, test findings, and response to care as evidenced by the facts. When a discordance of clinical data and documentation in the medical record exists, the CDI specialist is charged with the responsibility to bring clarity to the record.

This is where the query process comes in. It is what brings clarity to the record and allows it to be coded and reported accurately. A well-composed, compliant, and clearly understood query is an essential tool in the CDI toolkit. It must be employed with finesse, skill, a sound clinical foundation of disease processes, and a finely tuned aptitude for timing of the query.

As you have journeyed through this book and delved into the case studies, I hope that you've been challenged to explore different ways to approaching the clinical scenarios posed, that you have questioned yourself—perhaps even questioned some of the context in this book. I hope that you have been exposed to a broader approach that dared you to stretch and move outside your comfort zone in the process of exploring new approaches to reviews and query composition. Perhaps the "TRIC" approach will become solidly embedded in your query approach, ensuring that each query contains the essential elements of treatment, risk, and indicators that are clinically relevant, and lastly by the compliant question or request to the provider to clarify or further specify key components in the medical record.

Ensuring the integrity of the final coded medical record that serves as a legal scientific document is entrusted largely to the CDI specialist and the coding professional. With the clinical truth and integrity in our sights, we are partners in this endeavor to present the patient's clinical story.

REFERENCES

The Association of Clinical Documentation Improvement Specialists. (2018). *2017 Salary Survey: Salaries continue to grow, but participants are less optimistic than in the past* (Rep.). Middleton, MA: HCPro.

The Association of Clinical Documentation Improvement Specialists. (2018). *2018 CDI Week Industry Survey Report* (Rep.). Middleton, MA: HCPro.

The Association of Clinical Documentation Improvement Specialists. (2018). Case Study: CDI informaticist eases data woes. *CDI Journal, 12*(1), 20-21. Retrieved July 10, 2018, from *https://acdis.org*.

The Association of Clinical Documentation Improvement Specialists. (2017). *Developing Effective CDI Leadership: A Matter of Effort and Attitude* (Rep.). Middleton, MA: HCPro.

Cable, D. M. (2018). A*live at work: The Neuroscience of Helping Your People Love What They Do*. Boston, MA: Harvard Business Review Press.

Fries, K. (2018, February 8). 8 Essential Qualities That Define Great Leadership. *Forbes*. Retrieved June 30, 2018, from *www.forbes.com*.

HealthGrades. (2018). *Patient Safety Ratings Patient Safety Excellence Award™ 2018 Methodology* (Rep.). Denver, Colorado: Healthgrades Operating Company.

What is HL7 (Health Level Seven International)? Definition from WhatIs.com. (2015, June). Retrieved July 10, 2018, from *https://searchhealthit.techtarget.com*.